Real Men Get Prostate Cancer Too

2nd Edition
The Information You Want Your Doctor to
Tell You but You're Too Scared to Ask

Larry Axmaker, EdD

Health educator, psychologist, writer,
marathoner, and prostate cancer survivor (so far)
Co-author of *Cancer Clinical Trials*

Foreword
Tomasz M. Beer, M.D.

Grover C. Bagby Endowed Chair for Prostate Cancer Research
Deputy Director, OHSU Knight Cancer Institute
Oregon Health & Science University

Real Men Get Prostate Cancer Too

2nd Edition

The Information You Want Your Doctor to
Tell You but You're Too Scared to Ask

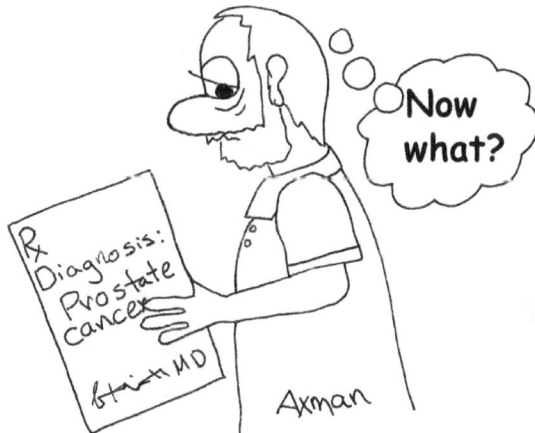

Larry Axmaker, EdD

Health educator, psychologist, writer,
marathoner, and prostate cancer survivor (so far)

©2008, 2012, Larry Axmaker

ISBN-13: 978-0-9854647-2-1

Olde and Graye Publishing

P.O. Box 963

Beavercreek, Oregon 97004

Phone (503)816-1876

Blog http://axman-axman.blogspot.com/

Cover: Lou Ann Baker, ladesignco.com

Production and Marketing: Concierge Marketing Inc.

Editorial: Write On, Inc.

PRINTED IN THE USA

10 9 8 7 6 5 4 3 2

Contents

Acknowledgments
2008 & 2012 Editions

Writing a book seldom happens without help from others. I have been lucky enough to receive help, suggestions, and support from a lot of good people. Words in a book aren't worth anything unless they make sense to those who read them. Thanks to those who have helped me to make sense.

For several years my wife, Carol, encouraged me to go ahead and do this. In addition to supporting me over my years of coping with prostate cancer, she also read, reread, proofread, and edited many written drafts along the way. And she still loves me after all these years.

Thanks to my sons and several old friends for reading various drafts and giving me encouragement and honest feedback.

And finally a big thanks to my friend the consumer-health writer and editor Sandra Wendel. She makes a living by writing and publishing monthly health content for a variety of business organizations. She took the time to walk me through the ins and outs of the editorial and publishing process, and she spent hours and hours getting this manuscript ready for printing. Her encouragement, recommendations, editorial talent, and occasional nagging made the actual publication of this book (twice) in this century possible.

Foreword

In the life of every man who stares down the barrel of a diagnosis of prostate cancer, there is always one day when the sun rises on a healthy man and sets on a man who has been told he has cancer.

What to do next is what every man hears a lot about. The doctors offer opinions and recommendations, friends deliver advice, sometimes welcome, sometimes less so. There are guides online and many books written by famous doctors, famous cancer survivors, and not-so-famous authors. There is lots of advice on what to do next. But how to do it is another matter.

Larry Axmaker, in his book Real Men Get Prostate Cancer Too, offers an invaluable how-to guide for living with the diagnosis of prostate cancer. Of course he talks about the principal choices men have to make and the answers they need to make good decisions about their treatment. But Larry has a keen ability to observe the human condition and offer commentary on it, which enables him to provide a unique guidebook for men whose peace of mind has been interrupted by the unwelcome intruder.

Prostate cancer is unusual among common cancers in that most men live with the diagnosis for many years. Recent data suggest that in the United States, five-year survival after a diagnosis of prostate cancer approaches 100 percent, and many men live far longer than that, often their full natural life span. Prostate cancer survivorship is a long haul. Doing it well is important.

There is a concept in medicine that draws a distinction between disease and illness. Disease is the physical condition, the bacteria that invade an organ, the cancer cells that grow out of control, the broken bone, or clogged blood vessel. Disease is a precise, biologic event.

Illness, on the other hand, is what human beings experience.It is the human condition in the face of disease. As an oncologist, every week I see how identical diseases lead to vastly different illnesses. Some men find ways to accept their diagnosis, co-exist with it, sometimes embrace it, put it in its proper place, but never let it win or let it sap and steal the vital energy that makes us fully alive.

These cancer survivors live their lives undeterred by their physical invader, even if some adjustments and accommodations must be made.Some are less fortunate and the disease devastates their ability to thrive. The illness these men experience is vastly different, even if the disease is largely the same.

Larry Axmaker's book is a how-to guide for being a survivor. Larry—a longtime prostate cancer survivor himself—brings into stark relief the hard choices, the challenges, and the losses men face. But he does all this with an unquenchable sense of humor and a spirit that simply cannot be diminished.

Tomasz M. Beer, M.D.
Grover C. Bagby Endowed Chair for Prostate Cancer Research
Deputy Director, OHSU Knight Cancer Institute
Oregon Health & Science University

You and Me and the Big PC

When you're diagnosed with prostate cancer, or any cancer, your life will change. You may not want it to change, but it will. Whether you're an optimist or pessimist, physically active or a couch potato, tall, short, heavy, or skinny, your mind will come back to your cancer again and again. Why me? Where did I go wrong? You'll think about it when you're driving, walking around the mall, watching TV, or even trying to fall asleep.

Constant worry can wear you down. That doesn't mean you can't help yourself, however. You can learn a lot about your cancer; find out what the treatment alternatives are, what they can and can't do, how you might benefit, and what actions you can take to make the quality of your life as good as possible for as long as possible.

This small book has been written by a guy who has prostate cancer for other guys who have prostate cancer.

What do you want to know about your prostate and prostate cancer?

What is a prostate?
What does it do?
Do I really need a prostate?

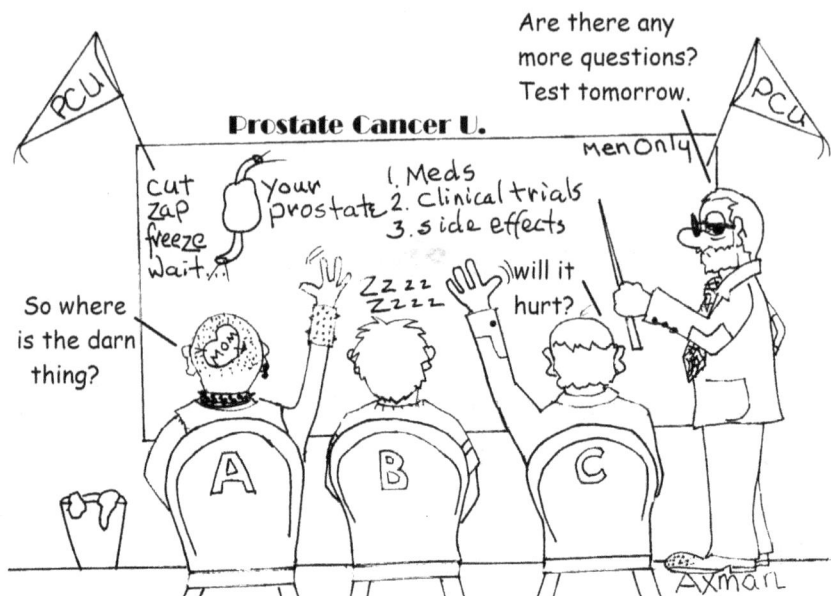

What exactly is prostate cancer?

Where does it come from?

Why do I have prostate cancer?

Who will help me?

What should I do?

What shouldn't I do?

What do I really need to know—bottom line?

There is a lot going on in the ever-changing prostate cancer world—research, treatments, clinical trials, lifestyle approaches, and personal choices. There is a constant supply of new information, better tests, new treatments, and other changes that can mean good news for you—and me.

Here's what I think I've learned: Real men (and most of us guys think we fit that definition) actually do get prostate cancer. A lot of us will, in fact. And whether it is diagnosed when we're 49, 63, or 87 there's a good chance it can be cured or managed. It works better if we do the right things—whatever those things may be.

And don't forget those wives, partners, and families who also have a big stake in this. They will do most of the worrying (research confirms this), make many of the medical appointments (common sense confirms this), provide the love and support we need (this defies common sense), and nag us until we follow through (thank goodness)!

And keep your sense of humor—it helps!

Larry Axmaker, EdD

1

The Macho Man and Prostate Cancer (It'll never happen to me, I said bravely)

Unless you have prostate cancer, think that you might have prostate cancer, know somebody who does, or were assigned to look through it by your spouse, you probably wouldn't be reading this book.

I hope you'll find some information, resources, support, and amusement as you thumb through these chapters.

Preventing, treating, or managing prostate cancer is a complex undertaking. There is NO single solution, but a lot of small steps may add up to a better outcome for you.

Your All-Too-Human Body

The human body—your human body—is an amazing and complex piece of engineering (as long as you don't believe everything you see in the mirror). Thousands of moving parts work together flawlessly (most of the time) decade after decade. Minor illnesses, injuries, and pains come and go. As you get older the aches and pains come more often and go away more slowly, but your body still works pretty well. Sometimes there are even unexplainable cures and improvements. Of course, if you're truly a macho man, you expect that.

There are, as you know, numerous parts in and on your body that can malfunction as a result of injury, disease, accident, and unknown causes. That's not even considering the normal aging problems created by such things as arthritis, failing vision, or hearing loss.

Your body can even function perfectly well without some of its original parts. Millions of people live long and near-normal lives after losing arms, legs, an appendix, tonsils, breasts, adenoids, testicles, a gall bladder, a kidney, a prostate, and other *expendable parts*. I hope that you aren't missing a lot of those parts, but life could certainly go on if they were missing.

And many parts you can't or don't want to do without can be replaced mechanically—knees, hips, arms, legs, and even a heart. You can be sure that more replacement parts are on the way. Living a long and high quality life with the help of spare parts is no longer mere fantasy.

Other body parts can be transplanted from donors— kidneys, liver, heart, lungs, retinas, and more (no brain transplants yet). Sometimes your own parts can be reattached if they are accidentally severed; fingers, toes, hands, arms, and legs have all been reattached successfully. In addition to a body that can survive the near-impossible, there is a worldwide scientific community that marches on and on to cure and replace what the body can't function without— usually at some cost, of course.

Then There's Cancer

Cancer may be the most dreaded word in the annals of health. It sounds devastating, fatal, and painful—even though that is often not the reality. Your body can fight cancer, often does so successfully, and you never even know there might have been a crisis. But sometimes cancer overcomes the defenses your body has implemented, and modern medical science may or may not have the answer.

My Story

Sixty-three cancer-free years is a good start—isn't it?

From my standpoint, men are supposed to be big, hairy, muscular, athletic, and tough. Being smart, too, would be a bonus. That is not necessarily an accurate description of me, however. We men typically consider ourselves to be indestructible and probably even immortal. Real men seldom consider their health and resist seeing doctors with a vengeance. And real men don't complain, either.

Recent enlightening events in my life, however, have suggested to me that we men are actually relatively fragile beasts. Don't tell my hairy, masculine friends I said that.

I started my intimate relationship with prostate cancer in 2003. I thought it would be a short encounter—it wasn't.

As a part of each chapter I'm going to share MY particular experiences with diagnoses, doctors, side effects, emotions, treatments, resources, second guesses, macho pursuits, good times, bad times, The New York Times, and even more. These passages will be easy to skip over if you wish—but I hope you'll take a look.

Prostate Cancer

Twenty or 30 years ago I didn't hear much talk of prostates let alone prostate cancer. Nobody talked about it and many people had never even heard of a prostate. How many people do you know who still call it a *prostrate*?

In recent years, however, we've all been hearing about prostate problems a lot more frequently (if you've been paying attention).

TV, magazines, newspapers, and the Internet tout cures for enlarged prostate, pills for erectile dysfunction, and tests for prostate cancer itself. Times have changed. Does it mean that there are more prostate problems than in years past? Probably not—but there is more awareness and publicity, and you're getting older and more likely to have a prostate problem.

About one of every three cancer diagnoses for men is prostate cancer. One in 10 male cancer deaths is from prostate cancer. This is a big deal if you're male. There's a lot to know and think about. You may have to make some life-altering decisions—now or sometime in your future.

What is it? Where is it? What can go wrong?

The prostate is a walnut-sized (some say crab apple size) gland located just below your bladder. Women do not have a prostate (that's good for them).

The prostate helps to control the rate at which urine flows out of the bladder and through the urethra. It does this with the help of muscles in the prostate that surround the urethra.

The prostate also plays an important role in sexual activity. The prostate gland makes a whitish secretion that collects within the prostate and is released into the urethra during ejaculation. This secretion helps the sperm move through the urethra. This fluid comprises about a third of the seminal fluid and gives the ejaculated fluid its whitish appearance and helps sperm swim toward any available eggs—or wherever.

The very thin nerves that allow men to achieve an erection run down each side of the prostate.

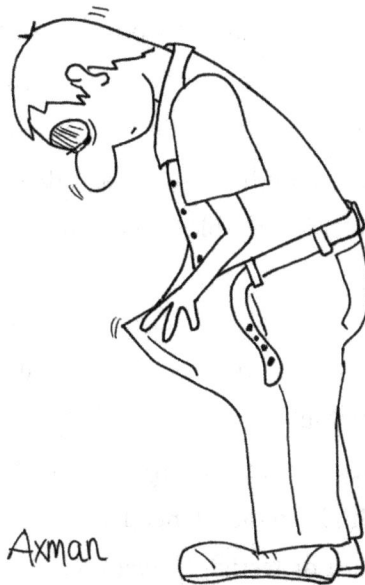

So, small and insignificant as it seems, the prostate serves some very useful functions. But unless there is a problem, you'll never even know it's there. There is no way you can see it, feel it, or even know for sure you have one without some medical assistance.

BPH

For most men, the prostate increases in size with age, usually after age 45, but it varies. The condition is called benign prostatic hyperplasia (BPH). Sometimes it's not so benign. As the prostate enlarges, it can squeeze the urethra, restrict urine flow, and make it more difficult and sometimes painful to urinate. Your bladder has to work harder to push urine through the urethra and in the process can become thicker and not empty properly. This increases the risk of pain, frequent urination, and increases your risk of urinary tract infection (UTI).

If you feel as if you have to urinate too often, especially at night, but can't always go or can't go very much, you may have a partial blockage—your doctor can find out for sure. In most cases this is a treatable problem. In extreme cases your urethra may become almost completely blocked or you can develop a serious UTI. These conditions need immediate medical attention. There are several treatments that can reduce blockages. BPH is not prostate cancer.

Prostatitis

Prostatitis is an infection of the prostate gland. It is common, painful, and treatable. There are several types of prostatitis, and most of the time antibiotics are the treatment of choice. The symptoms are similar to BPH: frequent need to urinate, difficulty urinating, pain in the urethra or testicles, swelling, pain during urination, and sometimes fever or chills.

If you are experiencing any of these symptoms, or other discomfort in your lower abdomen and urinary tract, see your doctor. Suffering is not always necessary. Prostatitis is not prostate cancer either.

Cancer and Men

No man ever expects to get life-threatening cancer—or any kind of cancer. "It could never happen to me!" Many men would consider getting cancer a personal weakness or failure. In fact, over a lifetime, your odds of being diagnosed with some type of cancer are a whopping one in two! So, if your neighbor isn't the one—it's you. Cancer isn't really funny, of course, but a little knowledge, a positive approach, and a sense of humor can make a difference in your survival and your quality of life after you are diagnosed.

Just a few decades ago many types of cancer were considered

death sentences. Some types of cancer were never even diagnosed and treatments were limited. It is not uncommon for the human body to have cancerous cells growing in various places. Many times your own body overcomes the cancerous cells. Changes in diagnostic methods and treatment have occurred rapidly in recent years and have helped save lives and improve quality of life.

Having a cancerous (or malignant) tumor in your prostate is not usually fatal. It is when the cancer metastasizes (spreads) to other organs or the bones that the risks may become life threatening. Even then there are treatments and procedures and lifestyle decisions that can increase life expectancy as well as maintain your quality of life.

My Story

There are many diseases and life-threatening conditions that can affect us men—especially as we get older (which most of us intend to do). Heart disease is the major culprit. Cancer is a close second. Stroke, respiratory disease, diabetes, and others trail behind. But none of these is likely to happen to me, right?

In addition, there are those conditions like arthritis, back pain, and chronic headaches that can reduce quality of life while not being immediately life threatening. But you can mostly manage or ignore those things. That doesn't even take into consideration the decisions men make that result in accidents (like driving too fast or drinking too much). And I didn't mention activities such as jumping out of airplanes, climbing mountains, deep sea diving, racing cars, and other things men do to impress women (probably doesn't work anyway) and other big, hairy men.

In recent years I've talked to a lot of men of various ages with various stages of prostate cancer and a few doctors who treat prostate cancer. Everybody has his own story and understanding of what he should do or should not do and what treatments work best. It isn't always based on credible medical research, but it is always passionately believed. Sometimes it works.

When I started through the prostate cancer diagnostic and treatment maze, I discovered there was a lot I didn't know. I looked for accurate information and couldn't always find it. There were many contradictions in the available information—which "truth" was I supposed to believe? What is real? What is pure bunk? What is merely an educated guess? Does common sense count? I decided to look for as much reliable information as I could and put it in an easy-to-read format. Information that is considered reliable today may be discarded tomorrow. I have tried to focus on the information that may be supportive or helpful to the guy who is actually living with prostate cancer and needs to know as much as possible to make the best decisions.

Believe me, it still won't make decision-making easy. It could even make the decision process more difficult. But getting as much accurate information as you can is the best way to understand your options—at least it seems that way to me.

A Brief History of Cancer

Cancer, in its many forms, has been around as long as humans have existed (probably). The first descriptions of observable cancer (tumors) were found in Egyptian writings from more than 3,500 years ago. They described breast tumors and how they were treated. Early medical professionals cut out the tumors and cauterized the incision with a "fire drill." Ouch. They also wrote (in hieroglyphics) that cancer was not actually curable.

Hippocrates, the famous Greek physician (known today mostly for the Hippocratic Oath taken by all doctors that includes the phrase, 'first do no harm'), developed the descriptions and terminology we still use to identify and describe cancer and cancerous growths. Early Greek and Roman physicians noted that when tumors were removed, they often grew back. Cancerous tumors were considered incurable and usually fatal. Those views persisted for most of the next 2,000 years. In the Middle Ages the people who cut out the tumors were often also barbers.

In the 17th and 18th centuries the development of scientific research and treatment methods brought about more sophisticated identification and treatment of cancers. Tumors were removed when they were found and were easily identifiable. Autopsies (although illegal in some countries) provided surgeons with information about the nature of cancer and tumor growth. Most cancers were still not curable, and many types were not even identified unless an autopsy was performed.

The development of anesthesia in the 19th century made surgery less painful and increased the likelihood of surgical success. Improvements in the microscope allowed researchers to understand how cancer cells grew and destroyed healthy cells. Although cures were still rare, this was all good news.

Researchers have now identified more than 150 kinds of cancer. The many types of cancers may look different, grow at different rates, have different survival rates, and be found in different parts of the body. Some types have a high rate of cure, some are slow growing, some are almost always fatal, and others are unpredictable. In many cases there are no easily identified symptoms in the early stages. Some, like lung cancer, can often be avoided by making wise lifestyle choices. Others, like prostate cancer, can sometimes be predicted but not usually avoided.

A Briefer History of Prostate Cancer

The prostate has probably been around as long as men have been around, but is rather new to the study of anatomy and medicine. The first written description of the prostate is attributed to an Italian anatomist in 1536, but prostate cancer was not identified until 1853—more than 300 years later. Prostate cancer was initially considered a rare disease (little did they know) probably because the normal male lifespan was no longer than 40 or 50 years and most men died before prostate cancer was likely to appear or become life-threatening.

The first recorded medical treatment for prostate cancer was surgery to relieve urinary obstructions. Removal of the entire gland (radical perineal prostatectomy) was first performed in 1904 at Johns Hopkins Hospital. After surgery the patients were both incontinent (no control of urination) and impotent (inability to achieve an erection). Radical prostatectomy as it is currently practiced was not developed until 1983 and has regularly been improved—good news for every man who still has a prostate. Risk of incontinence and impotence has been reduced but not eliminated (these risks will, we all hope, be further reduced in the future).

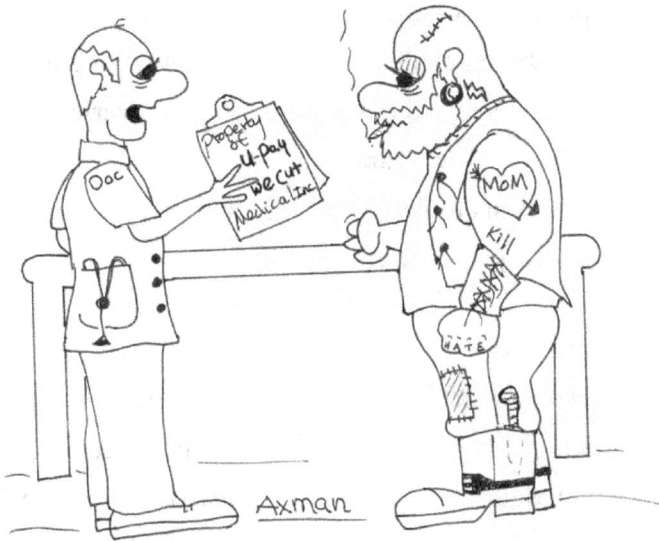

More Recent History

Recurring prostate cancer is often treated by neutralizing the effects of androgens that feed prostate cancer (mainly testosterone) and is called Androgen Deprivation Therapy (ADT). ADT slows prostate cancer growth and has been used for the management (not cure) of advanced prostate cancer since the 1940s. It is currently the only known treatment to significantly slow prostate cancer growth.

Radiation therapy kills cancer cells and was first used to treat prostate cancer in the early 20th century but the current form—various forms of external beam radiation—only became popular as stronger and more carefully controlled radiation sources became available in the last half of the 20th century when computers could help accurately map the areas to be targeted.

Although prostate cancer treatment is relatively new in the history of medicine, major changes and improvements have been made over a short period of time. In the 21st century, a man with prostate cancer has more options, a better chance of survival (according to medical research), and a better quality of life than his father or grandfather had just 30 or 50 years ago. All the approaches, discoveries, and research methods of the past few years lead directly to the advanced state of treatment that exists today. And there will be more advances—you can bet on it. You probably are betting on it.

Early Diagnosis—Late Diagnosis

Too many men don't find out they have prostate cancer until it's in a later and more serious stage—when there are noticeable side effects such as pain, fatigue, and weakness. If you're looking for a little good news, here it is. With regular checkups, early diagnosis, and some lifestyle changes, the five-year survival rate for early-diagnosed prostate cancer is almost 100 percent. That part has worked out for me. Almost 100 percent of me survived the first five years.

After skin cancer, prostate cancer is the most commonly diagnosed of all cancers. Approximately 220,000 men are diagnosed with prostate cancer in the U.S. each year, and there are about 32,000 prostate cancer deaths, second only to lung cancer deaths. These numbers will change slightly every year. So even though the numbers seem high, it isn't necessarily a death sentence. Most men survive prostate cancer—meaning they actually die from some other cause.

Where does prostate cancer come from? Nobody knows for sure.

Knowing that would make prevention and treatment a lot easier. There are lots of theories, studies, and educated guesses. There are links or relationships to genetics, lifestyle choices, and even a rare virus. But, at this time, the jury (or medical community) is still out. You will get it, or you won't get it. You'll be cured, or you won't. It's not quite that random, but prostate cancer is not easy to predict or to prevent. Older information is replaced by newer information on a regular basis. What is accepted as true today may be rejected next week. So it's not your fault you have prostate cancer—if that makes you feel any better.

Good Company

It should be no surprise that among the millions of men diagnosed with prostate cancer, there are many high-profile men who have or have had prostate cancer. Prostate cancer does not usually restrict physical and mental functioning. If you're diagnosed, you're in good company and have something personal in common with Bob Dole, John Kerry, Rudy Giuliani, Nelson Mandela, Sean Connery, Archbishop Desmond Tutu, Emperor Akihito of Japan, Colin Powell, Quincy Jones, Roger Moore, Sydney Poitier, Arnold Palmer, Joe Torre, Stephen Stills, Harry Belafonte, and Robert DeNiro.

None of these men is young, but at the time of printing all are alive, active, and getting on with their lives. Who could ask for more?

My Story

What has happened to me is not necessarily the same thing that will be experienced by you or any other man (that's probably good), but there will be parts that fit in with your experience.

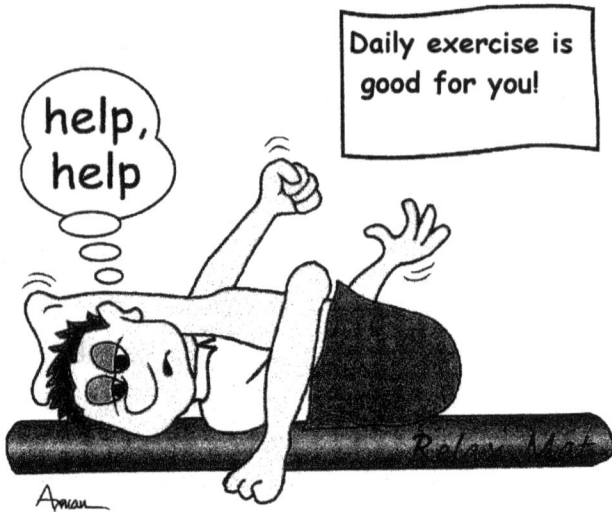

I'm lucky. For 63 years I had no significant diseases or illnesses: a bunch of broken bones (mostly from ill-advised manly pursuits) that pretty much mended themselves, a few minor surgeries, and some age-related conditions like arthritis, thinning hair, and an ever-expanding waistline. Excepting a strange passion for marathon running, my history wasn't much different from millions of other gracefully (if reluctantly) aging men.

The Costs

Treating prostate cancer is not cheap. The National Institutes of Health (NIH) estimates that the cost of treating prostate cancer in the U.S. exceeds $9 billion a year (that's $9,000,000,000.00). In addition to those costs is another $2 billion for treatment of BPH (enlarged prostate), prostatitis, erectile dysfunction, and urinary incontinence. This makes having health insurance very important in your decision-making process. Getting treatment is important, but it's also good not to go bankrupt in the process. Individual treatment can easily exceed $100,000 if the cancer recurs.

What should you be doing right now?

If you haven't been tested or retested recently, set up an appointment now. Your condition can change and there are frequently new studies and approaches and medications that may help you or that you may want to consider.

Get regular exams, whether or not you have been diagnosed. A DRE (digital rectal exam) and PSA (prostate specific antigen) test are relatively simple and inexpensive. If all is well, your doctor may recommend waiting a year for more tests—depending on your age and family history. No test is 100 percent accurate, but these tests are accurate enough to make them worth the time and expense.

The PSA Controversy

A large recent study concluded that most men do not need regular PSA testing. They say that it can lead to unnecessary treatment, stress, high costs, and physical risk. They claim there is no survival benefit—statistically. Another large study, conducted in Europe, came up with the opposite conclusion. It found a 20 percent survival effect.

For you, the individual, the statistics don't mean all that much. Either you won't get prostate cancer (statistically 0 percent risk) or you will (100 percent risk).

Many doctors believe the PSA screening provides information the doctor and patient can discuss in order to make good treatment decisions. If a tumor is fast growing, the PSA could help detect it and it could be lifesaving.

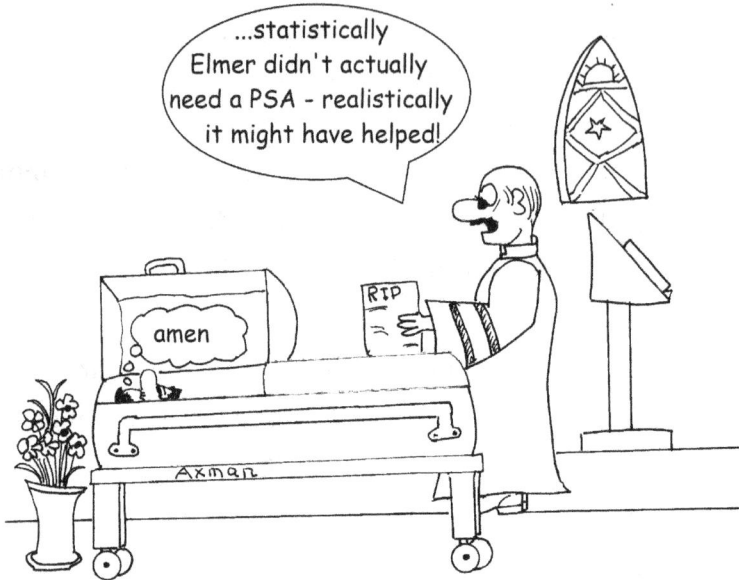

If you are tested and your PSA is higher than normal, you have a choice of what to do—more tests, active surveillance, look for treatment options, or do nothing. Knowing your PSA gives you options but does not require any specific action. Talk with your doctor—or several doctors and then decide.

You can't be over-treated for a prostate cancer that has not been detected. I, personally, would rather know than not know so my doctor and I together can determine what is necessary.

There is a good chance you will not remember to make an appointment, but your significant other probably will. A little time, expense, and discomfort now may lead to more good years in your future. If you don't smoke or chew tobacco, prostate cancer is the most common serious cancer risk you will ever have.

What about the risks you can't avoid?

Nobody gets prostate cancer before puberty, it is rare in young men, but it is quite common in older men. Those are the cold, hard facts.

Age—Your risk increases as you get older. That's bad and good. The bad part is that your risk gets higher and higher as you live longer and longer. The good part is that if you live to be 80 or more, you've survived longer than the average male lifespan already. Prostate cancer can be treated (or ignored) at any age.

Family history—Your risk of being diagnosed with prostate cancer is doubled if a close family member has prostate cancer. There's nothing you can do to change that, but it should motivate you to be tested regularly—starting now. The prostate health of your brothers and father does make a difference. Share your own test results with them and with your sons. Over your lifetime there is a one in six chance you will be diagnosed with prostate cancer. Some experts now say it's a one in five chance. If you are African American, your chances are increased. If your father or brother has been diagnosed, your odds change to one in two or three. If as many as three close relatives are diagnosed, your risk goes up to nearly 100 percent.

Hormones—Male hormones called androgens (specifically testosterone) are usually the food of choice that helps prostate cancer cells grow more quickly. Testosterone is also the hormone that causes masculine characteristics like a beard and low voice and allows sexual stimulation, sexual functioning, and reproduction. Depriving the body of testosterone will slow prostate cancer growth, and it will also reduce or eliminate sexual functioning.

Race—The risk of prostate cancer is highest if you are black, lower if you are Caucasian, and lowest if you are Asian. At this time, there is no clear evidence as to why there are racial differences. It could be genetic, diet related, or something else. You can't change your race, of course, so you might want to look at cultural differences in diet and activities associated with racial differences.

Can you actually do anything to reduce risks or slow prostate cancer growth?

The American Cancer Society reports that when prostate cancer is diagnosed in the early stages, the five-year survival rate is more than 99 percent. The 10-year survival is 92 percent and 15-year survival is 61 percent. These rates will probably improve as treatment options get better—at least I'd like to think they will.

Many experts (but not all) recommend that you start cancer screening at age 50 if there is no family history, but your doctor may recommend starting sooner. Screening (a PSA blood test and digital rectal exam) takes just a few minutes. Screening won't reduce your risk of getting prostate cancer, but could help in starting treatment if you have an aggressive form of the disease.

Prevention

Some cancers can be largely prevented. For example, to prevent lung cancer, stay away from smoking or avoid inhaling secondhand smoke. There is a direct relationship between smoking and lung cancer. To prevent skin cancer, avoid direct sun and use sunscreen, especially when you're young.

No such direct cause and effect is associated with prostate cancer. Prevention is not nearly so clear cut. That doesn't mean there's nothing you can do or that you can't take actions that might make you healthier overall and possibly help prevent or postpone or slow down prostate cancer. Throughout this book you will find information about foods, vitamins, supplements, physical activity, and other lifestyle choices that could improve your chances when coping with prostate cancer.

Diet

Yeah, yeah, you know the drill—herbs and twigs, right? There is no doubt that a healthful diet can help keep you healthy and help in preventing some cancers. As a matter of fact, the experts say as much as 60 percent of all cancer (but maybe not prostate) could be prevented or postponed with healthy living choices.

Eating a heart-healthy diet is also a prostate-healthy diet. Low or moderate fat intake is a good start. Unsaturated fats, in moderation, are good for you; saturated fats aren't. Do what you need to do; manage your weight and keep cholesterol levels in line—even if it's with the help of medications. Choose whole grains, fruits, vegetables, and fish as your main courses. It's not all just about good food choices; you need to manage calories, too. Too many good calories will still increase your weight and cancer risk. Caffeine and alcohol, in moderation, have not been shown to increase your prostate cancer risk—you don't have to deprive yourself of all pleasures.

Exercise

You don't have to compete in triathlons, climb Mt. Everest, or bench press 400 pounds—unless you really want to. But a two- or three-mile walk every day would be good. Swimming, biking, tennis, volleyball, and even golf (if you can keep your stress level under control) can help. Lifting weights a couple times a week helps tone muscles and stop bone and muscle loss. Stretching a little before and after exercise is a good idea, too. Having prostate cancer shouldn't keep you from exercising.

Attitude Adjustment and Other Difficult Tasks

Change the things you can, accept the things you can't change, and learn to tell the difference. That's the crux of the Serenity Prayer. And it's probably good advice when you have cancer. Worry and stress won't help and just might increase your risks.

Because depression is so common in late-stage cancer, get help before depression gets to you. Talk to somebody, take medications if you and your doctor think you need them, and do things that make you happy. Cancer won't get better or go away just because you're angry or depressed about it.

Will this guarantee you stay cancer free or even greatly reduce your chances of getting prostate cancer? Probably not. It may, however, increase your chances of surviving with prostate cancer. With a five-year survival rate of nearly 100 percent, taking care of your overall health can make a very significant difference in how your prostate cancer develops and how your body copes with it. Many men with prostate cancer eventually die from heart disease or other health problems, not from prostate cancer.

Surviving prostate cancer is certainly preferable to not surviving. Everything other than dying gives you a shot at the good life (or at least a life). Do what you can and don't focus on what you can't do. Many men with prostate cancer live near-normal lives for many years. Consider what side effects you would be able or willing to endure. For example, wearing a diaper at 77 may be a better choice for you than being dead at 63 without a diaper. A positive attitude and the ability to adjust to change are associated with living longer and having a better quality of life. Don't forget the benefits of maintaining a sense of humor.

My Story

At the point in my life before I was diagnosed with prostate cancer I considered myself living the very good life. I was already too old to die young and too young to die of old age. My wife loved me. My kids didn't think I acted my age (not sure if that was good or bad). And my grandkids wished I would spoil them even more. My dogs and cats pretty much accepted me the way I am—as long as they got fed regularly.

With retirement somewhere in my near future and the Social Security system still chugging along, my wife and I planned a future of some leisure, travel, camping, running, reading, and writing the great American novel (this isn't it). The fact that I ended up with prostate cancer was a glitch in my cosmic fabric and might change some of those plans—or maybe not. The word cancer sounds so final and dangerous it can overwhelm everything else in life—but I don't intend to let that happen (could that mean I'm in denial?).

2

Let There Be NO Symptoms

Many diseases have obvious signs and indications that strongly suggest you should take precautions, make changes, or see a doctor. You get red spots with the chicken-pox, fever with the flu, rash and itch with poison ivy, and a stomach ache with indigestion. Pain, swelling, and discoloration are Mother Nature's way of telling you to start doing something or to stop doing something. You learned at your mother's knee that everything that needs to be treated gives you some visual, painful, or at least uncomfortable hints. In this case, Mother wasn't 100 percent correct.

Prostate cancer doesn't play by those rules—or any rules. Your experience with prostate cancer will be different from anything else you've ever experienced.

My Story

Do the right thing—or no good deed shall go unpunished.
I had known there was such a thing as prostate cancer for a long time, but I never actually imagined that I could be at risk. Real men don't see doctors, get sick, or have any health problems (although real women do see doctors and generally live longer).

Why should I worry? My lifestyle choices were always healthy. I managed my weight, ran thousands of miles, ate fruits, vegetables, whole grains, and thought pure thoughts— mostly. As far as I knew at the time, nobody in my family had ever died or had even been treated for prostate cancer. I knew some guys who had been diagnosed and treated, but that was them, not me. For the past 20 years I had regular exams, but that was mostly to keep my wife from yelling at me. And all my test results said I was OK, not to worry, of course. I imagined myself sprinting across the finish line at the Boston Marathon at age 99. It could happen you know.

Reading about the risks of prostate cancer; impotence, incotinence, pain, scars, stress, and dying, has convinced me to ... quit reading.

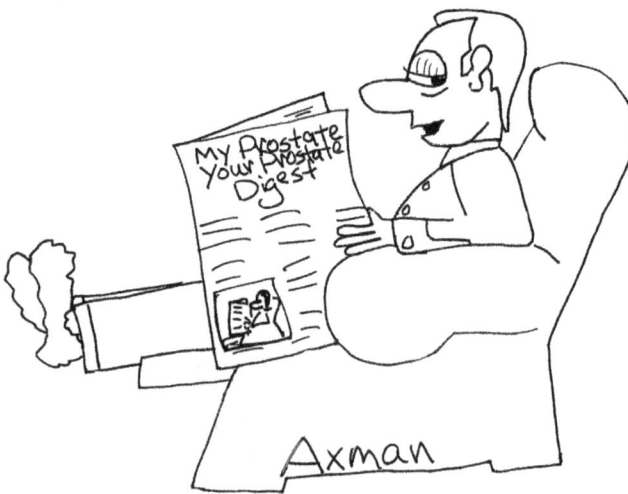

Prostate Cancer Q&As in a Nutshell (walnut shell, that is—same size as a normal prostate)

Q— What is the number ONE risk factor for getting prostate cancer?

A— Being a man who has reached puberty, but more likely is 50 or older. Your previous lifestyle may have some impact, or it may not. You may already meet the risk criteria in this category.

Q— What increases your risk of getting prostate cancer?

A— Getting older (something we all hope to do). A poor diet and a sedentary (no exercise) lifestyle may also be factors. And having a close relative with prostate cancer definitely increases your risk. Other factors may soon be identified, so stay tuned.

Q— If I am healthy, active, and have regular checkups, am I still at risk to get prostate cancer?

A— Yes (haven't you been paying attention?). Your risks may be somewhat lower, but the risk is still there. Men of all cultures, all sizes, and all socioeconomic levels are at risk. There are no (at least few) guarantees in life, especially when it comes to prostate cancer.

Q— When you have prostate cancer, do you feel pain in your prostate? Are there bulges that show? Is there blood in your urine?

A— Nope, not usually, and certainly not in the early stages. Prostate cancer can develop for years before any symptoms develop. That is one of the major problems in getting treatment. If you don't know it's there, you're not likely to get it treated. Read on.

Q— Is there anything that will indicate to me when I should get a prostate exam?

A— Common sense (which is not always so common), family history, and your doctor's recommendations.

Exams won't actually keep you from getting prostate cancer, but may or may not help you live longer if you do. It's not a perfect world. There are more treatment options available (including doing nothing) when prostate cancer is diagnosed early.

It's All Relative, Brother

Like many other diseases, there is a genetic link in the development of prostate cancer although the exact link is not yet understood. Has your father or brother been diagnosed with prostate cancer? If so, you should be tested at a younger age—ask your doctor. Err on the side of caution—find out. Finding out you don't have prostate cancer is better than not finding out that you do (at least that makes sense to me).

Because some cancers, such as prostate, do not have obvious symptoms in the early stages and nothing appears to be out of the ordinary, there is a tendency for men to put off exams; it's the macho thing to do. Male thinking often goes; "Why get checked out? If nothing hurts or looks strange, why push my luck and see a doctor?" For some men with slow-growing prostate cancer, this might be a perfectly safe and acceptable choice—for a while at least. But for others, putting off diagnosis could lead to an earlier death.

You may be thinking, "Hey, I'm a really tough guy and I'm in good shape. I run, swim, bike, lift weights, take vitamins, and eat tons of fruits and vegetables (and maybe a raw steak and too much beer now and then) so there should be nothing to worry about, right?" Right? Unfortunately, as you're now coming to realize, that's not exactly the case. Prostate cancer can happen to you without any known reason other than being a man. You could get hit by a bus next time you cross the street or be diagnosed with prostate cancer on your next visit to the doctor, but the bus is easier to see and to avoid.

To know or not to know—is ignorance really bliss? You already read about this in Chapter 1. If you weren't at least a little interested, you wouldn't be reading this.

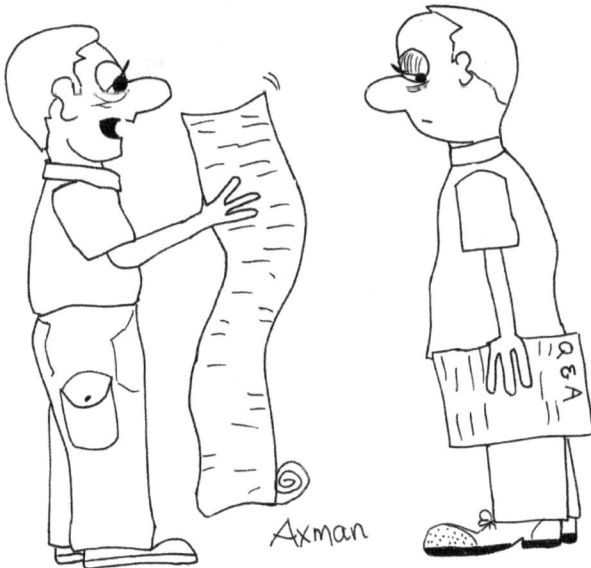

My Story

Life unfolds in strange and mysterious ways. Not only did I do all the right things (more or less), but during a moment of weakness in my mid-50s I agreed to participate in a seven-year prostate cancer study (clinical trial). It was a double-blind study with half the group taking an experimental drug that might help prevent prostate cancer and the other half taking a placebo (fake pill, sugar pill). There was a PSA blood test every year and periodic DREs. Everything in my exams came out normal—of course. I was not told (remember the double blind part?) whether I was taking the possibly-super-cancer-prevention meds or the plain, boring sugar pill placebo.

I found out in my final meeting with the testing organization that I had been taking sugar pills all those years. At least the price of the pills was right—and the exams were free, too.

At the conclusion of the study all participants were given one final PSA test and the option of having a free prostate biopsy. I might have preferred a free toaster, but that wasn't one of the choices.

A prostate biopsy involves taking multiple tissue samples from your prostate with a hollow needle inserted into your prostate through your colon near your anus. It's actually not as much fun as it sounds, but then it couldn't be. This type of procedure was nowhere on my list of fun ways to spend a summer afternoon but it WAS free. Why not, says I. More information is always a good thing. And anyway, I'm healthy as a horse, and prostate cancer is very rare in horses (I Googled it).

Preparing to See the Doctor

When you've had an elevated PSA score or other worrisome indication, take a little time for preparation before you see a doctor for your next prostate exam. What do you need to know and do? What information should you take with you?

- If you are seeing a specialist who is not your regular doctor, be sure to have copies of all your medical records. Your health history can make a difference in what happens next.
- Bring a list of all medications you are taking—including prescriptions, over-the-counter meds, vitamins, and supplements.
- Make a list of diseases and medical conditions your parents and siblings have, including prostate cancer, heart disease, other cancers, and emotional problems. It can affect your diagnosis and treatment options.
- Check with the medical office ahead of time to see if they want you to fast (not eat) before you come in—some blood tests require an empty stomach.
- Prepare yourself to hear good or bad news. In other words, go to the appointment with an open (and nervous) mind.
- Are you prepared to make treatment decisions if you are diagnosed? If not, what are you prepared to do? You probably won't have to make a decision very soon.
- Are you open to a variety of treatment options?
- Are you calm and patient enough to take a "wait and see" approach?
- Are you prepared to risk the side effects of the various treatments—such as incontinence or erectile dysfunction?

- Do you have adequate health insurance or some other way to cover the substantial costs of cancer treatment— often in the tens of thousands of dollars?
- Are you in good enough health to undergo surgery or prolonged radiation treatment?
- Ask questions and more questions. After all, it's your life.

However you prepare, just make sure you actually make an appointment and keep it. Most appointments with a doctor are uneventful and little new information is discovered. But you never know when you'll find out something that could change your life. So, like the Boy Scouts' say, "Be prepared."

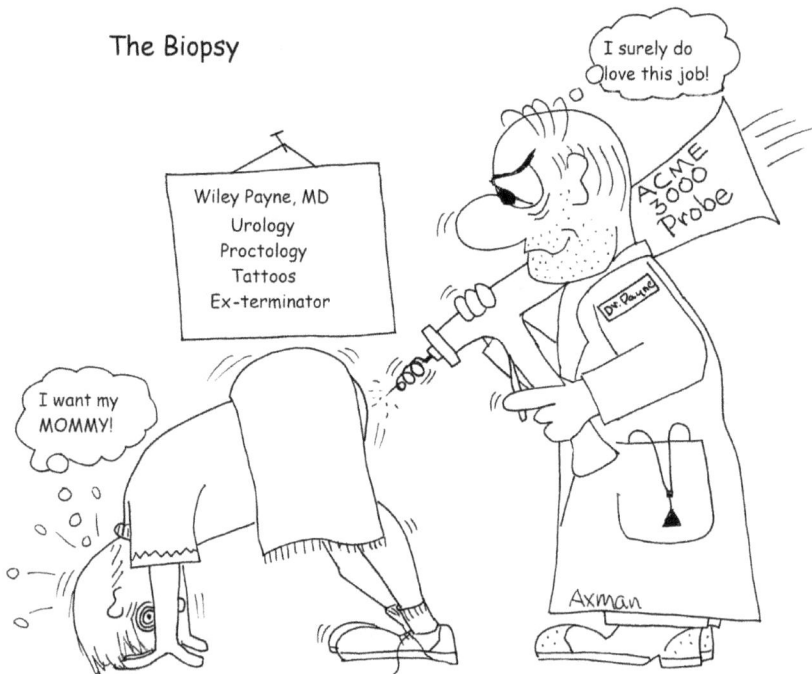

The Biopsy

My Story

So I showed up for the biopsy and was escorted into a small room with a padded table in the center. It all looked very sterile and medical. I felt a little nervous.

The biopsy rules, as explained to me, required me to remove my pants and lie on a table in a fetal position hugging my knees. There were four other people in the room (a doctor, a nurse, and two young interns) watching intently as the doctor in charge inserted some sort of medical device into my anus. This was certainly not one of the most dignified moments in my life. But it was free I kept telling myself. All in the interest of science.

A TV monitor on the wall showed the doctor where my prostate was and guided him as he carefully (I hoped) pulled the trigger to send hollow needles into my prostate to take samples. I couldn't see what was going on, but I could feel the sting of the needle each time it was inserted. It didn't take long and it didn't hurt much—just a "thunk" sound when the needle shot through the wall of my colon and into my prostate. They took six samples from me. I was certainly relieved when it was over.

I pulled up my pants and walked out into the August sunshine. I confidently drove home with my convertible top down and my thinning hair blowing in the breeze. I promptly forgot all about my adventure. As far as I was concerned, I was healthy, strong, and ready to attack old age like a bull in a china closet.

Fate, kismet, and divine intervention. The day after the

biopsy, I received a letter from the sponsors of my seven-year clinical trial thanking me for my participation and congratulating me because my last PSA showed that I was prostate-cancer free. Whee. I really wanted to believe them.

You've guessed what's coming next, right? Sometimes it doesn't take much to ruin your day, turn your world upside down, and change your life forever. For me it was the innocent-sounding ring of my phone. Three short days after my biopsy I got a phone call from the medical clinic that had conducted the biopsy. A disembodied voice said, "Dr. W,(the same urologist who took my biopsy samples) says to tell you, 'We need to talk..' That's all."

Those are words you never want to hear from your wife, mechanic, stock broker, or doctor. I felt like someone kicked me in the stomach, or lower. And of course I imagined the worst—whatever that may be. So I promptly made an appointment to "talk."

3

Those Dreaded Exams—
DRE, PSA, and Biopsy

Information about prostate cancer and checkups shows up in magazines, newspapers, on the evening news, your friends talk about it, and there are all those pop-ups on your computer screen. But a really determined man can always try to ignore it all.

Most guys would probably do almost anything to avoid being poked, prodded, or punctured by a doctor, even though he knows he should have his prostate checked—and why. And if he really doesn't know, some middle-aged woman will tell him. Whether you're 50, 65, or 80 could make a difference in your attitude toward exams and tests.

Is This Going to Hurt? Maybe. Probably

"But nobody in my family has ever been diagnosed with or died of prostate cancer or any other cancer, so why would I need an exam? Surely I'm not at risk."

A DRE should be a normal part of your annual physical if you're over 50, but that can vary from doctor to doctor. Your wife or significant other has finally made an appointment for you to be screened and you're trying to come up with two or three good reasons not to go. You have been threatened with dire consequences if you don't show up, so ...

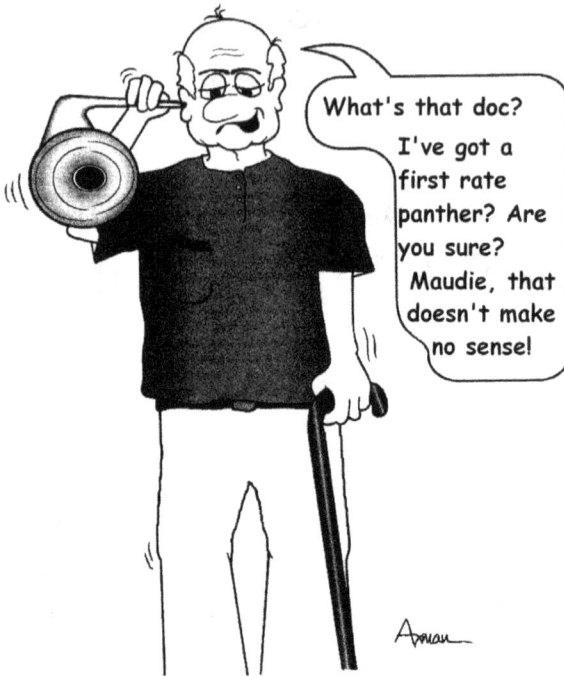

DRE—Dr. Jellyfinger Is Your Friend—Really

The most common prostate exam is called a DRE—short for digital rectal exam. It isn't much more pleasant than it sounds. The digital part refers to a doctor's finger (in a rubber glove, of course) and the rectal part is all about you.

After you are suitably attired in a backless hospital gown, or maybe you just drop your pants and lean over an examination table, your doctor puts on a rubber glove, dips a finger in some sort of lubricating jelly, inserts the finger into your anus and, through your colon, pushes, rubs, and probes your prostate to try to feel any irregularities, lumps, or swellings.

If there are irregularities, more tests might be needed. A lump or irregularity doesn't necessarily mean you have prostate cancer—sometimes (as Sigmund Freud might have said if he'd thought of it) a lumpy prostate is just a lumpy prostate. And, even if there isn't a lump, there could be cancer. Cancer or not, you're getting some useful information.

The DRE is not really painful, but it is definitely uncomfortable. You will feel a strong urge to urinate but can't and don't. The exam lasts only a minute or two (although it may seem longer). This test has been around for a long time and works well as a general diagnostic tool when the doctor is skilled and especially when there are lumps to detect.

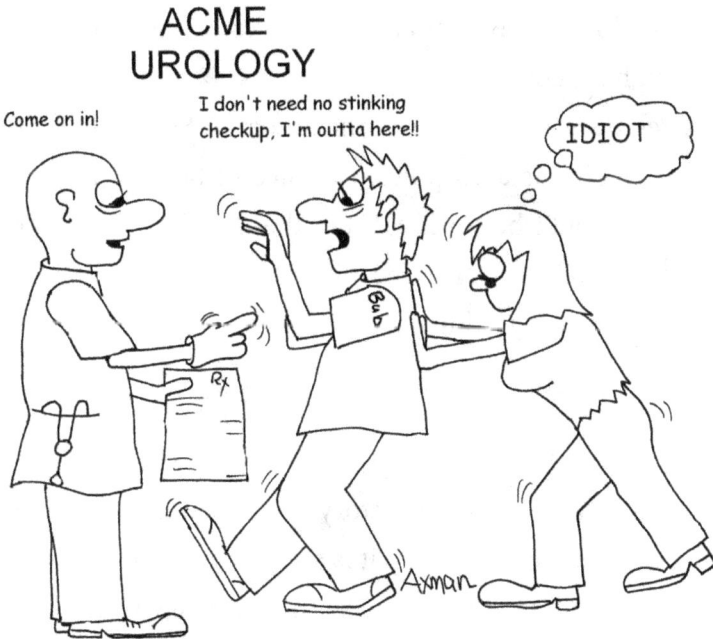

PSA—Just a Little Blood

The PSA (prostate specific antigen) test was developed more recently than the DRE. It is done by taking a blood sample that is examined under a microscope. Not to worry—the sample is from your ARM. It can take anywhere from 20 minutes to two weeks to get your results. The test results are usually reported as nanograms of PSA per milliliter (ng/ml) of blood. Although that may seem very technical and complicated, the results will be reported to you as a simple number such as 2.3, 5.4, 16.8, or 846. It can be as low as 0.0 and there is no upper limit.

If you are younger, you want the score to be 2.0 or less. Zero is always the best number.

If you are 55 or 60, 3.5 to 4.0 may still be considered marginally normal unless it has increased significantly since your last test.

Scores higher than 4.0 can indicate an increased prostate cancer risk (some doctors say that any score over 2.5 in men under 50 is high enough for concern).

PSA tests are about 85 percent accurate. So a test that shows a normal result has a 15 percent chance of being a false negative (meaning, it could be positive). On the other hand, a PSA of 8.2 could also be a false positive (meaning, it could be negative). Medical science isn't perfect yet, but you already knew that.

Biopsy—This Involves a Long, Hollow Needle and Is Not Going to Be Much Fun

Remember my free biopsy story in chapter 2? Here is a more detailed explanation. Although it is the least pleasant of the prostate exams ("pleasant" and "prostate cancer" are rarely referred to in the same sentence), a carefully conducted biopsy is usually the most accurate test. It can be done in a doctor's office, and little or no anesthetic is usually needed. You will need to remove clothing and kneel or lie in a fetal position on an examination table.

For the most common method of biopsy (called a transrectal biopsy), a hollow spring-loaded needle is inserted into your prostate through the wall of your large intestine (colon) just inside your anus, and small prostate tissue samples are removed—one at a time. Usually six to 10 (or sometimes more) samples are taken from carefully selected sections.

Your doctor will probably use ultrasound (using high frequency sound waves to construct an image of the prostate that can be seen on a TV monitor by the doctor) to be sure the needle is inserted in just the right place and at the right depth. The procedure may be slightly painful—like a bee sting every time the needle is injected into your prostate. Each sample is carefully tagged to make sure the exact location of the sample is known.

The samples are then checked under a microscope, and, if there is a tumor, its size and rate of growth can be determined by highly trained pathologists and technicians. You won't know your results for several days. When you get the results, they will be reported as a number called a Gleason Score.

Another method sometimes used to sample prostate cells is called a transperineal biopsy. A thin needle is inserted into the prostate through the skin between the scrotum and rectum. The sample is then checked by a pathologist.

Prostate Cancer Grades

When a biopsy determines that you have a tumor, the next step is to determine if it is cancer and if the cancer is a slow-growing or fast-growing form. Cancer cells vary widely in shape and size. Some cells grow aggressively and others may not. The pathologist identifies the two most prominent types of cancer cells and assigns grades.

Thinly sliced tissue samples are studied under a microscope, and cancer cells are compared with healthy prostate cells. The more the cancer cells differ from the healthy cells, the more aggressive the cancer is determined to be, and the more likely it is to spread quickly. The most common cancer grading scale yields a score of between 2 and 10, with 2 being the least aggressive form of cancer and 10 the most aggressive. It is called a Gleason Score, named for the doctor who invented the method. These numbers are helpful in determining which treatment option (if any) is best for you.

The type of cancer cell that is most numerous in your biopsy gets one of the five grades. The type of cancer cell that is second most numerous also gets a grade between one and five. For example, your primary grade (the most numerous type of cancer cell) could be graded a 4 (on a scale of 1 to 5), and your secondary grade (second most numerous type of cancer cell) given a grade of 3 (on a scale of 1 to 5). These two numbers are added together to determine a total Gleason Score. In this case the total is 7.

The lower the Gleason Score, the better your prognosis.

- Gleason score of 2 to 4 is considered low risk, slow growing, and not likely to threaten your life at this time. Scores in this range are usually not considered dangerous and no treatment may be recommended.
- Gleason Score of 5 to 7 is considered moderately aggressive and suggests that further analysis may be needed before treatment decisions are made. Treatment is usually recommended, but is not always considered immediately necessary.
- Gleason Score of 8 to 10 tells you the tumor is fast growing and considered high risk. There is a significant chance that the cancer will spread or has already spread, and most doctors will recommend that treatment should be started immediately.

My Story

So we talked—or he talked and I listened.

My wife and I arrived early for the dreaded "we need to talk" appointment, filled out all the proper papers, insurance information, disclaimers, and then waited nervously in a room filled with others who were also waiting nervously. Just about everybody in the waiting room was as old and worried looking as I felt. I wondered what their story was, but I didn't ask.

Finally it was our turn. Dr. W greeted us warmly, commented on the warm weather, and then, looking properly solemn, told me my recent biopsy indicated there was a tumor—a pretty big one as prostate tumors go—about the size of the end of my thumb. It was cancerous. He had slides, graphs, and charts to prove it and showed us a larger-than-life-sized model of a prostate (complete with tumor) and all the adjacent organs. I was impressed. I even got to touch it.

Stages of Prostate Cancer

The stage of a cancer helps the doctor determine how far the cancer has spread. The stage of tumor growth helps determine what treatment may be recommended. Prostate cancer left untreated has a tendency to spread to your lymph glands and bones. There are several ways of designating stages; the ABCD method and the TNM method are common. There are several possible stage designations, and your doctor can explain exactly what your staging designation means in practical terms.

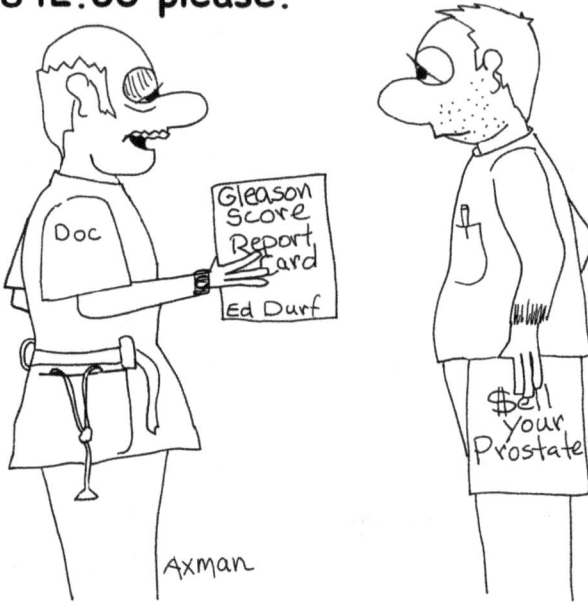

The National Cancer Institute uses a four-stage system.

Stage I—cancer is restricted to the prostate. It cannot be detected by a digital exam or by imaging. The tumor is very small.

Stage II—the tumor is larger but still contained within the prostate.

Stage III—the cancer has spread beyond the prostate to nearby tissues.

Stage IV—the cancer has spread to lymph nodes, the bladder, rectum, bones, liver, or lungs.

When your PSA is way too high

Whenever you have a checkup, you hope your PSA is low and has not increased since your last test; 1.3 would usually be just fine,

4.2 gives you pause, and 10.7 usually means a biopsy and possible treatment. But what happens when you get a PSA number that doesn't even seem humanly possible?

Every year thousands of men find out, often with their very first PSA test, that they have a level of prostate cancer that cannot be cured by surgery or radiation or any other first-line treatment. It is not impossible for a PSA score to be 1,000, 1,500, or even 2,000. That can mean the cancer has spread to lymph nodes, bones, and organs throughout your body. Certainly it means more tests—right away.

If your PSA is actually that high, it doesn't mean there is not treatment—just not a cure. It means that prostate cancer could be the cause of your eventual death. Modern androgen deprivation therapy (ADT) treatments can lower PSA readings, help manage pain, and improve quality of life as well as increase length of life. Chemotherapy has also been used to reduce pain and prolong life in very late-stage prostate cancer patients. And there are clinical trials that may be looking for new participants with your symptoms to try promising new treatments (see chapter 8 for more specifics).

My Story

Several cancer specialists had looked at the biopsy slides and all agreed with the findings. In my mind I could see a line of white-coated pathologists with long white beards all nodding solemnly in unison. My Gleason Score was 7, high enough to be serious.

Dr. W told me I had some choices to make. I wasn't going to die tomorrow or any time soon, but the tumor wasn't going to stop growing or go away by itself. Damn! He didn't pressure me, but calmly discussed options including surgery and radiation. He believed surgery to be the best option. He was a surgeon. His surgical success record was pretty good. He didn't mention active surveillance as a possible option.

How would I deal with this rather unpleasant information? How should I deal with it? How would you? My confused brain went through some rapid stages and changes. My mind, such as it was, raced through at least half a dozen scenarios in the space of a few seconds.

- *This is obviously a big mistake; has to be sloppy lab work, inexperienced doctors, or a greatly overstated diagnosis. There's really not a thing wrong with me. I'm as good as ever. I'm outta here! Bye, Doc!*

- *To hell with all the medical stuff. If it's true I'll just go on living my life the way I always have and let the chips fall where they may! It's my life, after all. Eat, drink, be merry, and die in my sleep, in a 200 mph car crash, while climbing Mt. Everest, or jumping out of an airplane and forgetting my parachute.*

- *Oh my God, I'm going to die! I'd better get my affairs in order (whatever that means) and say my goodbyes to family and friends. What clever quote should I choose for my tombstone? "He didn't find the answer to his prostate cancer" maybe.*

- *It's not fair. That stupid doctor should have found this years ago. Or maybe it's bad genetics; I inherited all the wrong genes. Of course it could be because of pollution and global warming. But it is certainly not MY FAULT!*

- *I need to do something now, right now! Maybe I can start treatment today or tomorrow. Cut it out, freeze it, radiate*

> *it, beam it into space, or something. But just do it!*
> - *Calm down, dude, take a deep breath, look at the alternatives, get professional help, and then do something rational and effective and final. No hurry. OK, that sounds a little better.*

One Is the Loneliest Number

Numbers, statistics, general trends, percentages, and average survival rates are great if you're reading about somebody else's cancer. When it comes to your cancer, the only number that makes any difference is *one*. You're the one. What happens to you, how you feel, and what you do may not have much to do with what happens to 249,000 other guys. At this point you're focused on you. I was focused on me.

Every Man Has a Different Story

Here are five short sketches showing how prostate cancer affected men I know in very different and sometimes unexpected ways and what choices these men made and are making. The information is true; the names and places have been changed to protect the innocent.

David owned and operated his own business. He was married and had two grown children. He ran, biked, swam, ate a vegetarian diet, and had regular health checkups. He considered himself as healthy as humanly possible. At his annual checkup, age 52, his PSA score had doubled to 7.2. He was sure he was too young for prostate cancer, so he was immediately retested and there was a similar result. He then had a biopsy that concluded that indeed there was a cancerous tumor. Within weeks he had systematically checked out doctors and hospitals and made arrangements to have prostate surgery.

Two weeks after surgery he was already going for long daily walks and was back at work part-time. It was business as usual.

Ten years later he is active and healthy and his PSA is still undetectable. Everything worked out exactly as it should have. He is happy to have made the choices he did.

Herman, a 74-year-old retired school teacher, was living his sunbird dream—summers in the northeast and winters in Arizona. He ate healthfully, walked several miles every day, and kept his weight down. His father and two brothers had been diagnosed with prostate cancer some years ago and he believed it was mostly a matter of time before he too was diagnosed.

At his semi-annual checkup, his PSA had increased to 7.3 and his doctor recommended a biopsy. To nobody's surprise, there was a tumor. His Gleason Score was only a 5, however, indicating that the tumor was relatively slow growing. After a lot of consideration and consultation with his wife and other doctors, Herm decided to continue having regular checkups, but not undergo any other treatment unless there was a major increase in his PSA or the rate of tumor growth.

Five years later, the tumor still seems to be growing very slowly and his PSA has increased only a little. He intends to continue living the active life he always has. He sees no reason to undergo treatment, but is keeping his options open.

John was long retired when he was diagnosed with prostate cancer at age 82. He worked in his wood shop every day, grew a large garden every summer, and bowled three nights a week. He had undergone successful treatment for BPH some 10 years earlier and there was no indication of cancer at that time. The cancer seemed to be very slow growing. His doctors recommended checkups every year and no treatment unless there was a change in the growth rate. Most of the time he forgot that he had even been diagnosed, and it did not affect his life in any way he noticed. For more than 10 years his PSA increased slowly. There were no symptoms and he remained self-sufficient and active.

John was 92 when he died from causes unrelated to prostate cancer. His cancer was never a medical consideration. He was the perfect candidate for the active surveillance approach. John was my Dad.

Jim was tall, trim, athletic, and energetic. He retired from the military and chose to work in landscape design as a second career. He loved the outdoors and hiked, fished, and hunted in his spare time. At age 50 he suddenly started to lose weight and experience serious and sometimes debilitating pain in his back and joints. Several doctors prescribed pain medication, massage, spinal manipulation, and dutifully checked for diseases and infections. There was no PSA or DRE done during this time. For nearly a year he continued to get weaker, lose weight, and live with severe pain. Some days he was too weak to go to work. He feared he was dying. Finally, a doctor friend suggested he be tested for prostate cancer.

At his first-ever prostate exam he was told his PSA was more than 1240. That's right, 1240. The cancer had spread to bones, lymph nodes, and organs. Jim's oncologist immediately started him on several Androgen Deprivation Therapy (ADT) drugs and his PSA almost immediately began to fall—after several weeks it was down to 400, then in just a couple months down to 50, and eventually dropped to 15! His back pain was also dramatically reduced.

There was no cure at this point, but Jim and his doctors were able to manage his symptoms for a while. He regained some strength and started gaining weight after the first several months of treatment.

The symptoms slowly came back and he lost his battle with prostate cancer within a year.

Dan was healthy, fit, active, and upbeat. He, his wife, and their two children were active in their community and in their church. He dutifully had exams every year, including a DRE and PSA. There was no indication of prostate cancer or any other cancer in his family. He was confident that he was at very low risk.

Everything was normal for many years, and then when he was just about to retire at age 65, there was a sharp increase in his PSA. A biopsy confirmed a rapidly growing prostate tumor.

After some consultation with family and friends, Dan opted for surgery.

His recovery was rapid, and within months he was back to his normal routine. Four years later he still tests cancer-free. He continues to live an active life with particular attention to exercise and a healthful diet.

My Story

You should always get a second opinion, I've been told—so I talked to another doctor. Same results. "Yup, it's a tumor and you should do something about it." This could NOT (or should not) be happening to me, I was indestructible. Other guys get tumors. I run marathons. My thoughts drifted toward self-pity. Phrases like "why me" and "not fair" and "life sucks" came to mind. It was hard not to be negative, even though I knew it wouldn't help. I already knew that life is not fair, of course.

I could choose to do nothing, tempt fate, and maybe lead a relatively normal life for a few years; even quite a few years.

This initially sounded pretty good—just carry on normally until something really serious happened like falling over dead. Active surveillance is an accepted treatment method—especially in older men (never considered myself in that category before) with slow-growing tumors. But Dr. W said I was young in terms of prostate cancer and my tumor appeared to be growing rather quickly. Bummer.

4

What Are THEY Going to Do to ME? Treatment Options for Every Man

One or more of the tests you reluctantly endured indicated the strong possibility that you have prostate cancer. And more tests were done—probably a biopsy. And it's true. You, along with several million other men, have prostate cancer. What should you do? Do you have to do something right now? Do you have time to ponder a decision? Inquiring minds want to know!

When There Is a Tumor—Even a Small One

You need to know that all prostate tumors (unlike all men) are not created equal—not that you have a choice of which type you grow. You may have a tumor or growth that turns out to be small or slow growing. That would be good news. But, in fact, many prostate tumors eventually grow to the point they become a threat to your health.

Even if the tumor is designated malignant, there are different growth rates and other factors you need to consider. Some tumors grow very slowly; others very rapidly. What the doctors find out through all the tests will have an impact on the choices you and they will need to make. The cancer can be

- **Local**—the tumor is completely contained in the prostate.

This is the easiest of all malignant tumors to treat. Cure is very possible—even probable. Maybe no immediate treatment is even needed.

- **Regional**—cells from the tumor are growing in the areas just outside the prostate. This will change the way the cancer has to be treated. But cure or successful treatment is still possible.

- **Metastatic**—cancer has spread to other parts of the body such as lymph glands, organs, and bones. Treatment is necessary to slow growth. While treatment is possible, cure is not—at least at this time.

You'll get lots of medical and nonmedical advice from well-meaning family and friends, but you're the one who will have to actually make a decision. Do your homework and take your time. You will learn that doctors specialize in specific treatments and will probably recommend the treatment in which they excel. So which doctor you talk to will affect the advice you get. That's a no-brainer. Knowing and trusting your doctor is a plus. You have many choices of doctors as well as several treatment options, or the option of choosing not to have treatment. Having a lot of options sounds great, and you may feel as if you're really in charge of your life. But it could also be confusing.

Ask Your Doctor

Whatever the diagnosis, you will probably want as much information as possible, and you have every right to expect clear and complete explanations from your doctor. The doctor may not know all the answers, but you should be able to get most of the information you want. Good, accurate information can result in better treatment choices down the line. But it helps if you can ask the right questions.

These questions are a good start:

- What is the likelihood that my tumor is encapsulated (confined to the prostate)?
- Do I need more tests? Why or why not? What tests?
- Do I need treatment now or can I wait a few months, or even years?
- What are my chances of cure or long-term remission?
- Is the cancer likely to come back later?
- Could I need additional tests or treatment later?
- Based on my age, clinical stage, grade, and overall health, what is my expected five-year survival rate? Ten year? Fifteen year? (Do you really want to know?)
- Would I survive just as long without treatment? If not, how long?
- Where should/can I get a second opinion?
- If you choose surgery, how many procedures has your doctor done? How many this year? Last year?
- What procedure does the doctor recommend? Why?
- What are my risks of incontinence or impotence?
- Should I change my diet and exercise regimen?

Ask for all explanations in common terms (not doctor speak) that are easy to understand. Ask for clarification of anything you don't fully understand. After all, it's your prostate and you're paying for the doctor's time. There are NO stupid questions when it comes to making decisions about your life.

My Story

Deciding on decisive decisions.

Being told I had a cancerous tumor growing in my prostate was a bit of a shock (actually this is meant to be an ironic understatement—it was a major catastrophic shock). Maybe I'll wake up in a sweat and laugh nervously about my bad dream. Maybe it's all a mistake. Somewhere in the back of my brain I knew it could happen, but I never really thought it would. Did they mix up the reports and some poor guy someplace else is really the one? If only. Whoops, that's not a very charitable thought.

There were a few treatment options to consider—radiation, surgery, freezing, radioactive seeds, active surveillance, and others. What's a guy to do? There was ample time to talk, read, meditate, cogitate, and worry. I managed to do all those things—over and over. These kinds of decisions suck.

After some of the initial mental numbness had worn off, my wife, doctors, and I discussed options. There wasn't any pressure from my doctor to decide right away, but I'm not a very patient person, and I wanted to get it (whatever it was) over with as soon as possible. According to most of the information I could find, the two most promising and available treatments that could—and probably would— cure me were surgery and external beam radiation. And my insurance would cover either treatment. So far so good.

Nobody knows what the best prostate cancer treatment is, although there may be a best treatment for you depending on age, stage, grade, and other factors. But you're unlikely to ever know which treatment that is without doing some homework. The good news is (good news may not be the right term here) you can usually take weeks or months to make a decision without increasing your risk. Be sure the decisions you make are those that make you feel most confident.

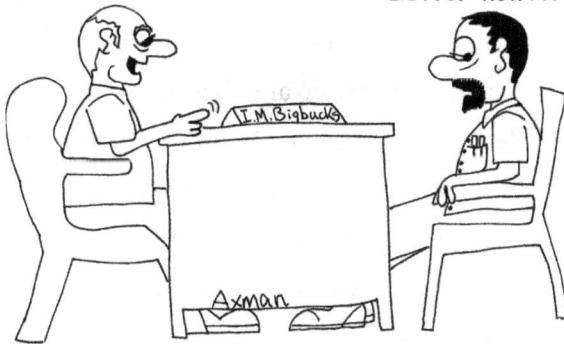

The Most Common Treatment Options

Because there are numerous treatment methods, individual preferences, and differences in the skill sets and availability of doctors, you'll want to know as much as possible about all the major treatment methods. The information that follows is just a start.

Active Surveillance

In cases where the tumor is small and/or growing slowly or the individual is quite elderly, treatment may be postponed as long as the cancer is not spreading or doesn't become life threatening. In some situations the man with the tumor decides to wait and see. In other cases treatment might pose a greater health risk than waiting.

With this approach, your doctor will most likely recommend a PSA and DRE at least every six months and biopsies every six to 12 months. This is most often used as an option for men older than 70 and those in poor health before diagnosis, for example, a man with congestive heart failure.

If You Choose Surgery

It's called radical prostatectomy. The medical rationale is this: Remove the prostate and surrounding tissues and everything is OK.

Surgery is a major decision and has some significant risks. It requires a skilled and experienced surgeon who can remove the prostate gland, resection the urethra (so you can urinate when you choose to and stop when you choose to), and save the nerves that allow you to have an erection (a good result, but not actually necessary for recovery or survival). The more surgeries a doctor has successfully completed, the better the overall results you can hope for. Practice does make perfect for a surgeon.

Surgery works best when the tumor is totally contained within the prostate. You and your doctor won't know that for sure before or maybe even after the surgery. You will be putting an important part of your life in your surgeon's hands—literally.

As a result of surgery, you will have a long scar from your navel to your pubic bone (radical retropubic prostatectomy) or an incision between your anus and scrotum (radical perineal prostatectomy). The surgery will take from two to four hours. These are the two most common surgical procedures.

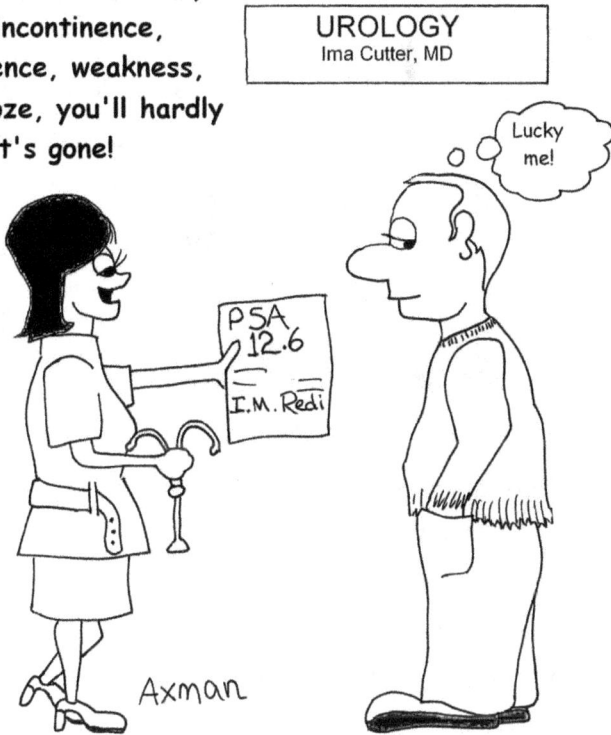

Other than the scar, pain, incontinence, impotence, weakness, and ooze, you'll hardly know it's gone!

UROLOGY
Ima Cutter, MD

Lucky me!

PSA 12.6
I.M. Redi

Axman

Some prostatectomys are done by cutting several small holes in your abdomen through which laparoscopic radical prostatectomy is accomplished with inserted tubes and the help of a small TV camera. New laparoscopic surgery techniques can result in a smaller scar and a more rapid recovery. You might even have a robot (possibly named R2D2, C3PO, or HAL—or not) to help in the procedure. Robotic-assisted surgeries are becoming more common.

Surgery will require you to spend several recovery days in the hospital, go through several weeks of at-home recovery, and weeks or months spent in diapers while your newly rebuilt (resectioned) sphincter heals and increases in strength. It may take several months or longer to become more or less sexually functional again—if at all.

Long-term incontinence risk is real, but relatively small to start with—in the 3 percent to 5 percent range with an experienced surgeon. But after five years the risk of some level of incontinence can rise as high as one in three. And, on a very practical note, whatever the overall percentage risk is, if YOU are the incontinent one, it makes the risk 100 percent for you. The statistics don't mean much when you're concerned about YOUR functioning. It either works or it doesn't.

Many thousands of men have adjusted to the unpleasant reality of some level of incontinence. It often seems to be a better option than doing nothing and dying sooner than you might without the treatment.

Impotence (no erection) is a larger risk—up to 50 percent. It doesn't take much damage to those thin nerves growing on your prostate to result in impotence. Many men have some ED issues before treatment. Little blue pills (and some in other colors, too) and other techniques and devices might help later. Both impotence and incontinence can get worse in the years after surgery—as is the case with some other treatment choices.

My Story

My wife and I finally reached a consensus. Surgery was the best choice for me—I think. Reaching a decision was a bit of a relief and I was sure it would be the last prostate cancer decision I would ever have to make. Surgery was quick and would remove the offending tumor. It's called a radical prostatectomy—the name itself is kind of frightening. A calmer name like safe prostate removal or insignificant small tumor surgery might have inspired more confidence. But I'm not in charge of creating medical terminology—yet. The decision was made; and to quote Shakespeare's Julius Caesar, "The die is cast" (I always wanted to say that).

Then along came the obligatory medical discussion about incontinence and impotence. This was the first time in my life I had ever seriously considered either one of those unpleasant possibilities. I couldn't let myself believe that either was a real possibility for me. It is hard to accept that next week I might not be the man I think I am today. So I tried not to think about it. Trying NOT to think about something almost guarantees that you WILL think about it. Oh well. I had strange dreams for a few nights.

So then what? Did the doctors think the tumor was contained? Yes (it actually was not). How soon should the surgery take place? How long should I wait? Once the decision was made, sooner seemed better than later. So I scheduled it for the earliest it could be—as long as it took to donate two pints of my own blood—just in case the surgery sprung a leak (it didn't). And I added an extra week to run another marathon—who knows, it could be my last one (it wasn't).

Having a month or more to think about the surgery could have had a calming effect on me (it didn't), but I didn't change my mind either. I couldn't imagine just waiting to see what was going to happen—even though that may have been a reasonable short-term decision and might have been the right decision for somebody else. No decision in life appears to be absolutely black or white. Mine was a very gray decision. I felt like a condemned prisoner choosing between hanging, electrocution, lethal injection, and being eaten by a tiger. I think I made the best choice for me at the time from a list of not very attractive alternatives.

Was surgery the right choice? Should I have waited longer? Maybe. Maybe not. Who knows? The wisdom of treatment decisions often becomes clear only in hindsight—one of life's little mysteries. It would be a year before I'd have any real answers, and even then it might only be a partial answer.

Medical consensus says you have about a 70 percent chance of being cancer-free for up to 10 years after surgery. That's good news, in general. But you need to be mentally prepared in case you happen to be in the other 30 percent. The numbers and percentages may help you in making a final treatment decision but won't guarantee you'll be cancer-free the rest of your life. Some recent studies give a slight edge to surgery over other methods in the long term. The likelihood of recurrence is very slightly lower with surgery as a first treatment.

If You Choose Radiation

Radiation treatment is popular partly because it doesn't involve surgery—no blood, no stitches, no pain. The medical rationale is this: Zap the tumor and it will eventually die. Probably. Radiation damages the cancer cells it hits and they gradually die. The normal, healthy, and useful cells around the cancer cells also die. In theory, the cancer cells die and do not grow back. The good cells that die do grow back. Radiation works best with younger men—those under 60 (it's true that in prostate-cancer talk, 60 is considered young)—who have an encapsulated (totally contained within the prostate) tumor.

With external beam radiation treatment, high-energy x-rays will kill cancer cells, especially if they are concentrated in a tumor. Your radiological team will take many x-rays, MRIs, and CT scans prior to your treatment to pinpoint exactly where everything is. You may even have several tattoos put on your backside to assist in aiming the big machine that delivers the radiation. Improvements are being made in the process and newer techniques are better at pinpointing exact areas to be targeted.

A computer program helps determine the exact spot or spots where radiation is to be focused. You lie very still on a table, likely in a partial pre-formed cast to minimize movement, and the x-ray machine with carefully aimed beams moves around you shooting short bursts of radiation into the tumor, or where they think the cancerous cells might be (if the tumor has already been removed). The results are cumulative—a little more radiation is administered each day.

Treatment requires numerous radiation sessions over weeks or months. Radiation can cause some side effects such as rash and burns on your skin, loss of body hair in areas radiated, and possible damage to your bladder, colon, and other nearby organs. There's no getting away from the possibility of side effects.

You will probably feel weak and tired for at least a few weeks during and after the radiation treatments. Some men feel nausea right after treatments, but it usually doesn't last more than a few hours and often doesn't continue after a few weeks of radiation.

Incontinence and impotence risks are about the same as with surgery. That's good news or bad news depending on which side of the statistical barrier you fall. With radiation, both incontinence and impotence can get worse over time. This may sound a bit grim, but you need to consider the side effects whenever you make treatment decisions. Risks and all, most men will eventually decide that doing something is better than doing nothing.

If You Choose Radioactive Seeds

The medical rationale is this: When small radioactive seeds (up to 125) are inserted, by needle, into the tumor, they will kill the cancer cells. Seed implantation (called brachytherapy) is usually used with low to moderate risk patients. There is no incision or freezing or external radiation, and recovery is rapid. Higher risk patients may receive seed implants plus external beam radiation—the idea being that the more the tumor is zapped, the better the chances of killing all malignant cells.

There are two types of brachytherapy: permanent and temporary.

- **Permanent Brachytherapy**—Radioactive seeds/pellets are inserted into your prostate. They give off a low-dose radiation over a period of time. The radiation emitted by the seeds generally has a half-life of about 60 days (meaning that the effect of the radiation is greatest during that time). Once inserted, the seeds stay in the prostate forever but don't seem to cause any long-term problems.

- **Temporary Brachytherapy**—In this procedure, the radioactive seeds/pellets are inserted into the prostate, but are left there for a very short period of time—usually about 15 minutes. These seeds emit a high dosage of radiation for this short period of time and then are removed. Three separate treatments is the norm.

The side effects of brachytherapy treatments are about the same as with other types of treatment. There may be a slightly lower risk of impotence with this method.

If You Choose Cryosurgery

The medical rationale is this: Freeze the tumor and it will die. Cryosurgery (or cryoablation surgery) can be used even after radiation is used as the primary treatment and the tumor starts to grow again. It is currently used less often than surgery or external beam radiation. Impotence and incontinence are common side effects.

In cryosurgery several hollow probes (usually six to eight) are inserted into the tumor and a very cold gas is injected to freeze it. The tumor is cooled to minus 20 to minus 40 degrees Fahrenheit (really cold), thawed, frozen again, and thawed again. Some nerve damage is common. The frozen cancer cells die. So do the frozen healthy cells around the tumor. At the same time the prostate is being frozen, warm saltwater is circulated through a catheter in the urethra to prevent it from being frozen.

Cryosurgery is used less often than other treatments, and long-term effects have not yet been fully determined.

Hormone Therapy (Androgen Deprivation Therapy)

Hormone or Androgen Deprivation Therapy (ADT) is the most common treatment when prostate cancer is advanced and considered incurable. It is often used in conjunction with other treatments to slow prostate cancer growth. It is also sometimes called estrogen therapy. It can be used as a first-line treatment when the cancer is first diagnosed at an advanced stage and has spread to bones and organs. In these cases the normal first-line treatments would not be effective. ADT neutralizes or slows the effects of androgens—primarily testosterone. Testosterone is a major food source for most prostate cancer cells.

In women, estrogen is a hormone secreted by the ovaries, which affects many aspects of the female body, including the menstrual cycle and normal sexual and reproductive development. It affects breast growth and other secondary sexual characteristics. A reduction in estrogen at menopause can result in hot flashes and other discomforts. Men who use ADT for a length of time may have some of the same physical effects that women have from estrogen.

ADT use can cause a change in the male shape and pretty much eliminates sex drive. But ADT often slows prostate cancer growth—sometimes for several years. It has been one of the most effective treatments for prolonging life. Side effects can include weight gain, breast growth, increased body fat, fatigue, hot flashes, and reduced HDL (good) cholesterol. You'll have to weigh the side effects against the effects of not using hormone therapy.

Prostate cancer, however, is adaptable and can mutate over time and eventually learns how to grow without testosterone. So this is not a cure.

Orchiectomy (removal of testicles)

The most effective way to reduce male hormone production is called orchiectomy (castration). This is the medical term for removal of the testicles, and this procedure reduces hormone production by more than 90 percent. Although effective, for some strange reason a majority of men are reluctant to undergo castration. Orchiectomy results in total and irreversible impotence and loss of libido (sex drive).

And, Finally, Chemotherapy

Chemotherapy has been used to treat cancer for many years and has proved to be effective for many types of cancer. A chemical cocktail is usually injected into the bloodstream or dripped from an IV bag. Fast-growing cancer cells (and sometimes other fast-growing cells like hair follicles) are targeted and killed.

Chemotherapy works best with cancers of the blood and lymph systems. It has not been used as much or as effectively with prostate cancer. It is often the treatment of last resort, when everything else fails. New combinations of chemicals have been able to extend life for those in the late stages of prostate cancer.

Chemo has had an unexpected benefit for me - I haven't had to shave or get a haircut for more than a year!

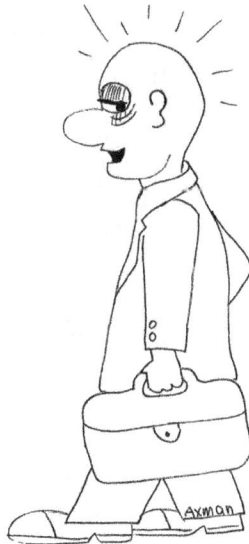

Chemotherapy drugs kill normal cells along with cancer cells and can cause side effects such as nausea and vomiting, hair loss, loss of appetite, fatigue, mouth sores, increased vulnerability to infection, and risk of bleeding and bruising.

Other Treatments in Use and Development

Linear Accelerator Radiation: The linear accelerator uses microwave technology (similar to that used for radar) to create high-energy x-rays. A portion of these x-rays is collected and then beamed into the tumor. The beam comes out of a part of the accelerator called a gantry, which rotates around you. You are lying on a moveable treatment table, and lasers are used to make sure you are in the proper position. Radiation can be delivered to the tumor from any angle by rotating the gantry and moving the treatment table. This treatment is expensive and currently available at only a few locations. Watch for more research about long-term results.

Proton Beam Radiation: Proton beam radiation bombards the diseased tissue (tumor) with protons instead of x-rays. Protons are positive parts of atoms that cause little damage to tissues they pass through but are good at killing cells at the end of their path. This means that proton beam radiation may be able to deliver more radiation to the prostate and do less damage to normal tissues that are nearby. Early results are promising, but a long-term advantage over standard external beam radiation has not yet been proven. Watch for new research information. This treatment is currently available at only a few locations.

Nothing, Nada, What Problem? (The do-nothing-just-now approach): Ignore it, do nothing, and plan no treatment. Prostate cancer often progresses slowly and can take years to become life threatening. This approach may be more common than you think, but is not always the recommended approach. Men who may wish to avoid the stress of dealing with the cancer treatment or are unaware of what choices they have may choose this option. This is not the same as when your doctors recommend an active surveillance approach. This is when you refuse or choose not to have any tests or make any plans.

The downside? By the time you get diagnosed or decide to take action, it may be too late to institute some or all of the standard treatments.

And Now a Few Kind Words About Impotence

ED (erectile dysfunction) or impotence is a common outcome in many if not most prostate cancer treatments. This may or may not be a serious problem for the men going through the treatments and their partners. Although you may experience ED, your libido and ability to achieve orgasm may not always be significantly affected.

There are several treatments that may be at least partially effective. Discuss all options with your doctor.

- **Oral medication (pills)**—can be effective if nerve-sparing surgery was used or another treatment method was used that didn't damage the nerves that are necessary to achieve an erection. It is the most natural method of achieving erection through sexual stimulation.

- **Intra-urethral suppository**—pellets inserted into the urethra work for some men. The procedure takes some training and has possible side effects such as penile pain.

- **Penile injection**—an injection into the penis expands the blood vessels and allows the penis to become engorged with blood, effectively causing an erection. It requires training to inject the drug and can cause pain.

- **Vacuum device**—easy-to-use way of drawing blood into the penis causing an erection. It can cause numbness or bruising.

- **Penile prosthesis**—there are several types of implants that are surgically inserted into the penis. These devices work when no other method has been effective. There is some risk of infection and the implant erection is permanent.

Support Groups

There are support groups for many diseases and conditions—everything from addictions and dependencies (everybody is familiar with AA, for example) to various types and stages of cancer. The number of prostate cancer support groups is growing as the number of men who are living with prostate cancer increases.

Many hospitals, senior centers, and clinics, especially in large urban areas, will have cancer support groups that meet on a regularly scheduled basis. The format will vary, but typically meetings occur monthly and the groups are rather informal.

Often the sessions will include an educational component—a cancer professional may be invited to share what's new in prostate cancer treatment, clinical trials, and other useful information. A member of the group may present new research findings or a film or DVD may be shown.

Most sessions include a sharing/discussion time. Talking about coping, concerns, what works, what doesn't, and whatever else is on your mind can help relieve stress. Everybody in the room knows what you're talking about; they all have the same condition to varying degrees.

Check with the American Cancer Society, your doctor, hospitals, senior centers, or other men who have prostate cancer to help find local support groups. Be wary of groups listed online or otherwise advertised that ask you for money to join or receive information.

5

Making the Best
of the Worst Choices

When you are diagnosed with any disease, you almost always have some choices to make. In many cases it is relatively simple; you will choose to do what your doctor recommends to cure or manage the malady. Pull that wisdom tooth (didn't improve my wisdom), physical therapy for the tennis elbow (never did play tennis very well), or arthroscopic surgery for that torn knee cartilage (or I could just limp).

When you are diagnosed with prostate cancer, however, the number of possible choices can be confusing, overwhelming, frustrating, and none of available options may be the choice you really want to make. Seldom is there just one possibility. Here is the dilemma:

> *You* have recently been diagnosed with a tumor in your prostate, and by now you actually know where your prostate is. You know the options—at least most of them. Your head may be spinning and it may be very hard to believe that you actually do have cancer.
>
> Your doctor has made recommendations and you have dutifully seen other doctors who also made recommendations, some of your friends have shared their recommendations with you, and unfortunately no two sources may have suggested the same treatment.

Now the choice of what to do or what not to do is really up to you and your health insurance carrier (many medical decisions rest heavily on those "bean counters" who control the medical insurance purse strings). Be absolutely certain the doctor and hospital you choose are covered by your health insurance. Treatment can be very expensive. Or be sure you have a healthy bank account.

Each possible treatment has its risks and advantages. Do your homework. Check out your doctor. Know before you start that there is NO guarantee of success. Feeling confident in the choices you have made before you start treatment is a good thing. That still doesn't guarantee success, of course.

Because prostate cancer often progresses slowly, there is almost always time to weigh alternatives, gather more information, and make a more or less educated decision. Age is a factor. Studies have shown that when men are first diagnosed in their 70s or 80s they are likely to eventually die of a cause other than prostate cancer. But when men are first diagnosed in their 50s or early 60s they are likely to live long enough for prostate cancer to become life threatening.

A recent mega-study (a review of 500 previous studies) came to the conclusion (or non-conclusion) that there is no definitive evidence to recommend any specific prostate cancer treatment. And other studies have shown that whether you have immediate treatment or even postpone it for months or years has little effect on the ultimate time of survival after diagnosis.

My Story

Cut me to the core, Doc, in my manly regions.

Believe it or not, major surgery was nowhere on my to-do list—or at least it was way down toward the bottom of the second page.

This particular surgery was more serious (and frightening) than any others I have had and the only one that could be considered even moderately life threatening. There had been the odd oral surgery, two arthroscopic shoulder surgeries, knee surgery, and various minor cuts and stitches and broken bones. But none of the previous conditions offered the possibility of being incontinent and/or impotent or even dead forever—however long that is. You never know what might happen next, but I wish I did. There are always major decisions to be made in life, even if none of the choices seems to be very pleasant.

Worst case ... I could end up incontinent and impotent. I kept telling myself that even if I had to wear a diaper and merely shake hands with my wife at bedtime, it was probably better than letting the cancer spread. If you consider yourself a macho guy, being impotent doesn't seem like a very good lifestyle choice, but modern science has discovered all sorts of pills and gadgets that could help. But none of those nasty side effects was likely to happen to me anyway. Not me!

All sorts of strange and unusual thoughts randomly straggled through my mind—"why didn't I ..." or "I should have ... " "I could have lived a better life" (couldn't we all). It all sounded kind of maudlin, like I was experiencing the soap opera version of my life. Cue the dramatic organ music (no pun intended).

I was still young after all—at least in my mind— my wife even accuses me of being childish sometimes. The best worst decision was to go ahead—and try to keep smiling (sort of). Doing what I had already determined was my best chance was some small consolation. And everybody I talked with was genuinely supportive. A lot of really great people wished me well, prayed for me, and shared their love and concern. That boosted my confidence and was even calming to me, but also made me feel a little guilty—I didn't really deserve all their goodwill. I discovered that in this stressful situation I had more support than I would ever have imagined. That was good.

The Risks—Revisited (just in case you forgot)

Incontinence (Small but real chance)

Most of the major prostate cancer treatments have a similar risk of incontinence. The sphincter muscle between your bladder and urethra that allows you to control the flow of urine is small and fragile. It doesn't take much to alter its functioning. After treatment—even years later—incontinence can occur or get worse. As men age, they can also become incontinent for reasons completely unrelated to prostate cancer—another of Mother Nature's dirty little tricks. You could end up in pads or diapers—which for most men would still be preferable to being dead.

Incontinence can certainly alter your activities, choices, and quality of life. On a more positive note, pads and diapers allow you to continue doing many or most of the things you need to, want to, or just enjoy doing. Even when your initial prostate cancer treatment is successful, your chances of becoming incontinent can increase as the years go by. In fact, however, for most men the risk of incontinence does not cause them to opt out of treatment.

Impotence (Greater and very real risk)

Most of the major treatment options also have a similar risk of impotence. It is a common side effect. Sexual functioning is not something that is required to live a more- or-less normal life, but most men would certainly prefer a life where sexual functioning is at least possible. You are constantly reminded of sexual functioning and erectile dysfunction by the plethora of TV ads and computer pop-ups promising that a certain pill will make you a whole man

Heads - Surgery
Tails - Radiation
Neither - ignore it!

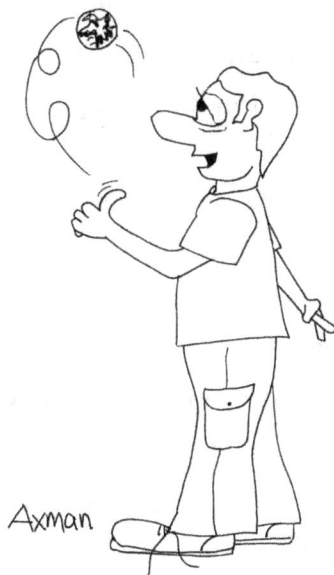

Axman

again. Maybe. Maybe not.

If the tiny nerves running along each side of the prostate are damaged by any treatment, it could be difficult or impossible to attain or maintain an erection. Are you willing to take that risk? The risks may sound very different to a 37-year-old than they would to a 73-year-old. Again, this is largely a quality-of-life risk. That won't make it any easier to choose.

Depression/Stress

"I could die." "I might die." "I'm going to die." Your mind is not always your best friend. The realization that you have a serious and possibly life-threatening disease can be a serious emotional blow. Something is happening to you that you can't completely control (men often like to be in control).

You may experience feelings of anxiety, fear of dying, a general feeling of lethargy or depression, anger, and you might feel terribly alone and isolated. You could become short tempered with those close to you or even withdraw and refuse to talk to them at all. Your friends and family might think you are pushing them away and they might be right. You may feel sorry for yourself, "It just isn't fair."

It is important for you and those you care about that you talk with your doctor if you have any of these concerns or feelings. Talk with your partner, friends, anyone you know who has survived cancer, or to a counselor. Many men who become depressed can benefit from counseling and medication, even if they have doubts. Depression, left untreated, can even lead to suicidal or homicidal behaviors. But, in most cases, the intensity and destructiveness of the emotions can be avoided or managed. Depression can be treated. This is a situation you can control.

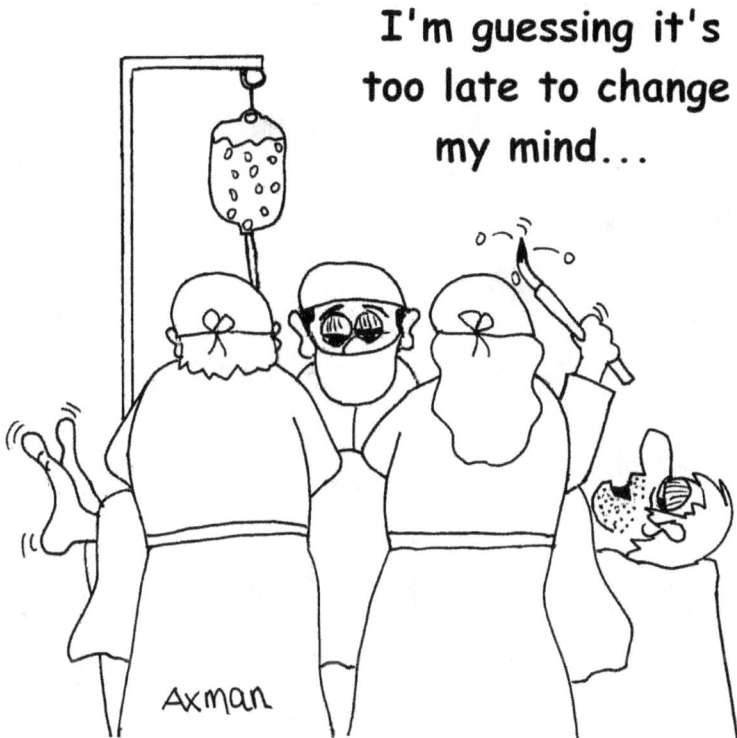

I'm guessing it's too late to change my mind...

Axman

Treatment Guarantees and Other Misinformation

No doctor can guarantee success. Medical personnel are expected to be upbeat, positive, and encouraging. They should not, however, guarantee success.

If your doctor tells you there is a 100 percent chance of cure, you should immediately go find another doctor. All treatment has some risk and there is also risk in choosing not to have treatment. But the reason you seek treatment is because you believe there is a greater risk in NOT having treatment. If you and your doctor determine that treatment would pose a greater risk to you than not getting treatment, don't do it. But in most cases, treatment of some kind will eventually be in your best interest.

My Story

All the medical personnel assigned to my surgery team were upbeat, smiling, friendly, calm, alert, wise, professional, and very supportive. But then I was paying THEIR salary and THEY weren't going to be prone on that operating table (not today anyway). They went through this every day with people a lot worse off than I was. My once-in-a-lifetime trauma was business as usual to the hospital staff. Maybe that's a good thing.

"They know what they're doing, they know what they're doing, they know what they're doing..." (Repeat as necessary, I told myself).

As my wife, son, and I walked into the hospital on that October day, those ironclad, confident decisions I had made two months ago seemed a lot less final now than they did then. I was at best nervous, and in fact more than a little terrified. What was I getting myself into? Was it too late to change my mind and run away as fast as I could? Probably. Here comes a smiling nurse now. Damn.

Not making a choice is still a choice. Doing nothing is still a choice. As time goes on, and you don't make treatment choices or start treatment, your options may narrow. Depression can keep you from making decisions until it may be too late for some options. Make a commitment to yourself to do everything possible to give yourself the best chance of survival and a good quality of life.

Humans are very adaptable creatures. Get the support you need to help you make logical and practical decisions. The choices you ultimately make may not be the same as the choices your neighbor or brother might make in a similar situation, but if you did your homework, your choices will probably be the best ones for you.

6

After the Fact—
Recovery Would Be Nice

Once you and your family and your doctor agree on a treatment and you go ahead and do it, there will be a mandatory period of recovery. When your body experiences trauma of any kind, it takes time for you to recover emotionally, gain strength, and get back to some semblance of normality again. You will never be exactly the same again.

Recovery time and discomfort can vary with the procedure you had and with individual differences related to age, general health, and fitness. Whatever the treatment, you will need time for recovery. Take the time you need.

My Story

I'm alive and well—at least most of me is.

Being prepped for surgery is not all that difficult. For a few minutes you just lie there and let somebody (or several bodies) shave and wash you (I was afraid to move in case they made a slip with the razor that would make the surgery unnecessary), put an IV connection in your arm, and talk calmly.

Although they talked calmly, I was not very calm at all, and my heart rate was off the charts. I felt exposed and vulnerable—

probably because I was exposed and vulnerable. Then the bags were hooked to the tubes and I was wheeled down some long hall (it certainly seemed long but all I could see was the ceiling) toward an operating room, or so they told me.

Surgery—no big deal! The surgery itself was easiest of all. As soon as they started that IV drip and told me to count backward from 99, I was out (unconscious) and remained so for more than four hours—they told me it was four hours anyway.

Somebody else did all the work; I was just the practice dummy. I never knew how many masked professionals were hovering over me during the procedure. When it was all over, I woke up very slowly and rather reluctantly in what they call a Recovery Room. But waking up after the surgery was definitely a plus—a positive first step toward recovery. I was pleased to be awake, although I had not actually planned for a different result. So far the plan had come together just the way it should. I love it when a plan comes together.

I gradually became aware of a series of tubes going into and out of various parts of my body, but there was no pain. Morphine is truly a wonder drug. After a while I recognized my wife and assorted children and started to remember who I was and why I was there. It was done—at least the bloody part of it. So, everybody, please just leave me alone and let me sleep. That twilight zone between being conscious and unconscious is rather pleasant. But it didn't last long—not long enough.

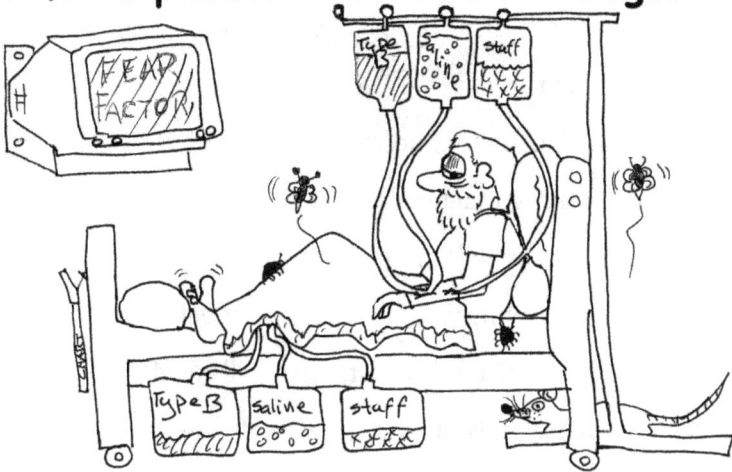

I have the no-frills plan... Each night they just switch the bags.

Time and Type of Treatment—Surgery

Surgery is the most invasive treatment, but also the treatment most often chosen.

Recovery Rule number one—It will take longer than you think it should and later it will hurt worse than the doctor said it would. It's a good thing treatment decisions are made before treatment. Some men would never agree to some treatments if they knew how they'd feel the day after. The day after part does mean that you're still alive, however. Look on the bright side.

Recovery Rule number two—After a week or two of tubes and bags, you will depend on Depends® (or another brand of personal absorbent undergarments). After surgery you will be totally incontinent for at *least* a few weeks. This is not an option. It almost always gets better, but the recovery time can seem lengthy and can vary a lot from man to man. It can be a frustrating time. Patience is a useful skill at this juncture. Impatience will not speed up the process.

Recovery Rule number three—If you feel good, strong, and healthy right away, you're probably not living in the real world and should refer back to rules one and two again; you may have received too much pain killer. Give yourself permission to take the time to heal. There's nothing macho about trying to do too much too soon. Everyone around you will understand.

Cancer surgery will have an ongoing effect on your body. You WILL be weak and tired. Your stitches will need time to heal. The muscles under the incision will also need time to knit. It will take weeks or months to start feeling more or less normal again. Some doctors tell their patients to expect to feel tired and weak for up to a year. Listen to your medical team. Don't do anything that will actually slow down your recovery.

My Story

It seemed that as soon as I was conscious, a nurse and her muscular helper encouraged me (there was not actually a choice) to get up (slowly) and go walking (actually shuffling and stumbling) down the hall—very slowly, with a foggy head, rubbery knees, and with bags and tubes dangling. Some bags dripped stuff into my body and others drained stuff out of my body. I hope they don't get them mixed up. It all balances out in the end, I suppose.

When Will It All Work Again?

Don't you wish. After surgery there will be a tube from your bladder, through your penis, and emptying into a plastic bag. Once you're up and around, the bag will be tied to your leg. Nobody else will even notice (much), but you will hear it slosh from time to time. Don't forget to empty it once in a while.

GUS embellishes a little bit...

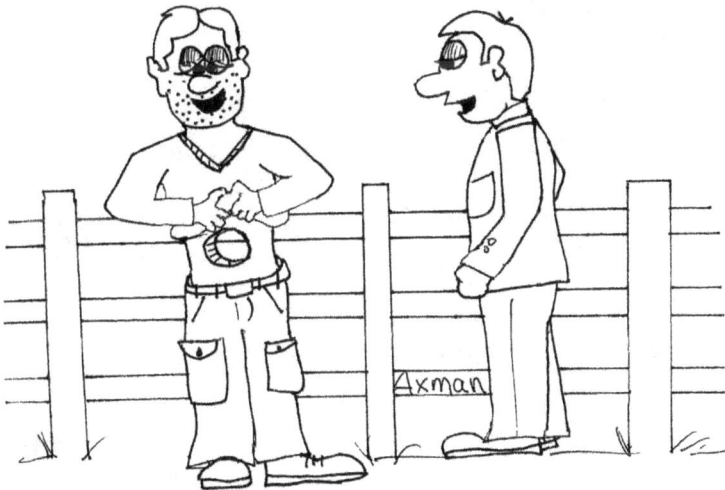

They had my prostate out in 15 minutes and I was home mowing the lawn in an hour...

Wow, I'm impressed! How soon can I get mine done?

The tube is usually removed in 10 days to two weeks. It is actually almost painless to have it removed, but you'll cringe (guaranteed) because you THINK it's going to hurt. Then you go into diaper mode. It could take two months or more before you can graduate to just a pad in your underwear. Several months later, if all goes well, you will not need any extra protection, but you will not likely feel the same urinary confidence you did before surgery. If your wife has been pregnant, she will understand the feeling. When you cough, sneeze, reach for something on a high shelf, or maybe just laugh, you might leak a drop or two. No big deal, but you'll notice.

As far as sexual functioning—you may be able to have an erection within a month or two, or never. There is no way to predict ahead of time how you will recover sexually. But, as mentioned several times already, there is help in the form of pills, devices, and even implants.

If you are able to have intercourse and orgasm, it will be different—dry with almost no fluid. There will probably be a little urine leakage. Sorry, guys.

My Story

Recovery was going to take a while. But right now I didn't much care—as long as the morphine held out. My morphine drip was on a timer with a button I could press to increase the drip rate up to the maximum amount allowed. As a macho guy who can withstand gobs of major pain, I figured I didn't need much of the morphine. But in fact I used every drop that was available. So much for my manly image!

Did they get all the nasty cancer cells? The doctor said he thought so and I sure hope so. There was no way to know yet. And I probably wouldn't know much for a few months or more. My tumor was gone, my prostate was gone, a large section of my urethra was gone, and I had a stomach full of shiny staples in a jagged row. But for the moment, I didn't feel all that bad, or good.

My high-tech hospital room was rather large, as hospital

rooms go, and I had it all to myself. With no outside window, there was no way to know if it was day, night, sunny, or rainy. It didn't actually matter much. Lots of people came to visit and brought flowers, balloons, and moderately tacky get-well cards. That was nice.

Later I realized that I didn't remember a lot of what happened for the first couple of days. Time seemed to be flying by—which may be the real curse of old age. They let me go home on the third day. Thank goodness.

I started feeling better right away. The first day home I walked around the house then the yard and within a week around the block. All this was done with a catheter tube running into a waterproof (hopefully) bag strapped to my leg. Slosh, slosh, slosh.

A week and a half after the surgery I attended a concert— the Simon and Garfunkel Farewell Concert. We got tickets long before I was even diagnosed and there was no way I was going to miss it. Nobody seemed to notice the bag on my leg. A couple of days later the catheter was removed by a smiling nurse who told me it wouldn't hurt. It didn't. A week after that the staples came out—that didn't hurt either. I was back at work in two weeks with a good supply of diapers in an athletic bag (I didn't call it a diaper bag). But all good things come to an end and I was out of diapers and into pads before I knew it (whew).

Three months after surgery I could run a few miles relatively pain free, I didn't have to wear diapers or pads anymore, my sexual functioning had returned more or less, and I felt pretty good. Could life get any better? Probably, but I wasn't complaining. I was still alive and confident I was cured! I was living up to the most optimistic post-operation predictions. I was the poster boy for prostate cancer recovery!

I ran a 50-kilometer ultramarathon on mountain trails nine months after surgery, just to prove to myself and to the whole world (which didn't seem to care very much) that I could do it. I had to stop and pee a lot, but I was relatively strong and in control, and I finished with the help of a patient running partner (my son). Was I back to normal or what? Woo hoo! There was nothing I couldn't do now!

Time and Type of Treatment—Radiation

Radiation is a popular treatment and has very different initial effects than surgery. There will be no scars, stitches to heal, or muscles to rebuild. You probably won't feel any particular effects from radiation at first.

As the radiation treatment proceeds for a week or two, you will likely feel tired, maybe nauseous, and may be bothered with rashes or burns from the radiation. Various medications, salves, and ointments can reduce the itching and pain. Ask your doctor and treatment team for their recommendations.

But after radiation is completed—weeks or months—you could find your ability to control urination gradually diminishing—just the opposite of the improvements you would expect after surgery. Bladder control and sexual functioning may initially be near normal but gradually get worse for a year or several years—then again they may not.

The damage from radiation is cumulative, and cells can continue to die for a time after radiation is completed. There is no medical model that predicts what will happen for each individual man. Once you go through a treatment, you will have to learn to cope with the side effects—as if there was a choice. And if the side effects are not what you expected, get help. There may be other reasons for the side effects or symptoms. There may be medications or exercises or devices that can help you.

Don't be bashful when you visit your doctor. Unlike your wife (wives see all, know all, and perceive all), your doctors won't know what you're feeling or thinking or experiencing unless you tell them.

Time and Type of Treatment—Cryotherapy

Damage from cryotherapy (freezing the tumor), like radiation damage, may show up gradually over time. Be prepared for ongoing and possibly worsening side effects such as incontinence and impotence. Frozen or damaged cells can die gradually and cause side effects to appear weeks or months after treatment.

7

Curses on You, Mother Nature! When Cancer Comes Back

My Story

Say it ain't so, Doc.

Fast forward one year after surgery. Post-operation PSA test number four. I was on a first-name basis with Dr. W by now and we discussed running, travel, kids and grandkids as well as my PSA.

Remember the "did they get it all" question? Well, apparently the answer was NO. Naïve me never really considered it might come back—what are the odds of that? (About 60 percent for all types of cancer over time—remember?) What did I do wrong? What did the surgeon do wrong? Probably nothing. Anyway, it doesn't matter who did what when cancer comes back. Blaming someone doesn't change anything. It's still your (or in this case, my) problem. And I definitely considered it a problem.

Although my PSA number was still very low, it had doubled each three months for four consecutive tests—way too fast and definitely not a good sign. Damn. Double damn (the complete original response was edited by the official text censor to keep this book's PG-13 rating). "Think positive," said Dr. W. So I did, "I'm positive I'm going to die this time." But that feeling, too, passed.

So now what? I could choose to do nothing and see what happened, or I could look for a Plan B. Remember the part about me not being very patient? I was all ears when Dr. W recommended additional treatment while my PSA was still low and the cancer easier to kill.

After a very short period of pondering the alternatives, the decision was this: We agreed Plan B would be radiation therapy. So, barely 15 months after my surgery I was sent off (actually downstairs in the medical complex) by Dr. W to see Dr. N. Radiation can be used as primary therapy or as a secondary approach, as in my case, to get the last remnants of those nasty cancer cells that somehow survived my surgery. I must be feeding them very well.

Thousands of American men (and even more worldwide) have cancer surgery every year. You probably know a few men who had surgery or another treatment. Most of us just assume that once something is cut out or properly zapped, we're cured. Did you ever hear of an appendix, gall bladder, or impacted wisdom tooth growing back? Me neither.

In the real down-and-dirty world of cancer, sometimes you're cured and sometimes you're not. The choice is usually not yours to make.

All those glowing and upbeat statistics about being cancer free and high survival rates sound great, unless you end up in group B—which includes all those who do get cancer again. Nobody actually volunteers to be in group B. Recurrence can be a greater emotional shock than the initial diagnosis. The first time you're diagnosed and treated, you're pretty sure you'll be cured. When it comes back, your mortality is in question. Do you throw a tantrum or blame or sue somebody? Maybe, but it won't change anything.

The medical term is biochemical recurrence, which simply means even though you had one or more types of treatment, the cancer is still there and still growing. In the U.S. more than 50,000 cases of prostate cancer biochemical recurrence are diagnosed each year. You're not alone brother, but that's a small comfort at this point. Prostate cancer is hard to completely eliminate, as you now know.

If you had a form of radiation therapy as primary treatment, then radiation would not be used for follow-up therapy. And if you had surgery as your primary treatment, there is nothing more to remove. Did you know that prostate cancer can exist even when there is NO prostate? Of course you do, now! You've heard about the numbers, percentages, and odds, but you don't think it will actually happen to you—unless you're a true pessimist and expected the worst all along. The tests must be wrong. So you have more tests. You always want to have another test.

There is about a 60 percent (or 70 percent or 50 percent depending on the research you read) chance that once you have cancer and are "cured," you will get cancer again in your lifetime—even if there is no measurable cancer after your initial treatment. Did anybody tell you that before your treatment? Maybe yes or maybe no, and even if they did you probably weren't listening. You were cure oriented at that time. In fact, there is no way to know for sure if all the cancer has been killed or removed. You can only wait, have tests, wait some more, have some more tests, and repeat.

It doesn't take very many cancerous cells left in your body to allow for recurrence or continued growth. It depends on your immune system, heredity, and probably more than a little dumb luck. One malignant cell may be enough (maybe it takes a few more than that but you get the idea). Cancer cells are pretty tough and resourceful and ruthless— but you already knew that, too.

Now What?

If you had surgery and the cancer returns, your doctor may recommend a series of radiation treatments. Whatever concerns you had with incontinence and sexual functioning will reappear. You may have already lost some functioning. You may well lose more functioning. In fact, you probably will. A 50 percent chance of impotence plus another 50 percent chance of impotence doesn't necessarily mean a 100 percent chance of impotence, but your odds diminish with each treatment. Whatever you've gone through and whatever functioning you've regained is at risk again. Take a deep breath and allow yourself the time to make the best possible decision.

My Story

Zap it!

After the obligatory phone call to my insurance company I decided to go ahead with external beam radiation (sounds kinder and gentler than radical prostatectomy, doesn't it?).

In the careful preparation for the radiation treatments, I was x-rayed, scanned, measured, and tattooed (really). The tattoos (actually just small, drab black spots spaced out on my backside) were used to guide and aim the radiation beams and then remain as a long-term reminder of the procedure, although I've never actually been able to see them. My wife tells me they're not much to look at. Or maybe it's just my backside that she thought was not much to look at.

A cast was made for me to lie on so nothing moved during the treatments. I would lie on my stomach, bare bottomed, on a big, flat, cold table and the large x-ray machine would move around me emitting short growling bursts of radiation that were carefully aimed at spots or areas where cancer cells might be. Without a tumor to aim at, the focus was on areas where the cells could be, probably were, typically hung out, or were last seen. Ain't science grand?

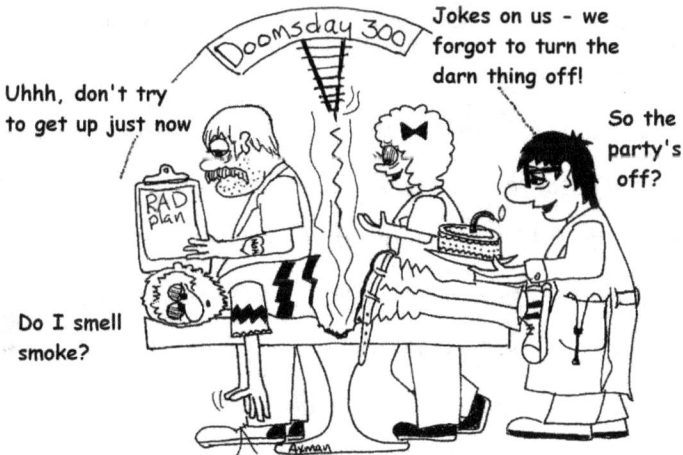

If you had radiation treatments initially and the cancer has not spread to the lymph nodes, organs, or bones, your doctors may suggest surgery. With surgery as your secondary treatment, you have the same risks as you would with surgery as a first option, plus the side effects you already have from the radiation therapy. Making a decision this time around could be even more stressful than the first time you went through it. The original treatment failed, the risks are higher, and it may be hard to maintain a positive approach.

My Story

The treatments themselves were short and painless. I went in five days a week for more than seven weeks. After the first week or two, I started feeling tired and run down and occasionally nauseous. This got better over time. There were, however, some other side effects such as radiation burns on my skin, mostly on my backside. My skin would sprout rashes, split open, and sometimes bleed. Sitting was no longer my favorite position. I used a lot of creams, salves, and lotions. They helped some.

The radiation beamed into my body was measured in RADs (units of absorbed radiation), and the oncologist determined how many RADs my body could stand each day and week and overall. A newer term used is Gray (one Gray is equal to 100 rads). You have treatments until you reach that limit determined by your radiation oncologist. So, eight weeks and 37 radiation treatments later, it was over again. And a month after that my PSA numbers dropped to the lowest measurable limit, again. The painful radiation burns started to heal, but the tender skin persisted, and a year later the bleeding still occasionally occurred for no apparent reason. I now understood references to being thin skinned.

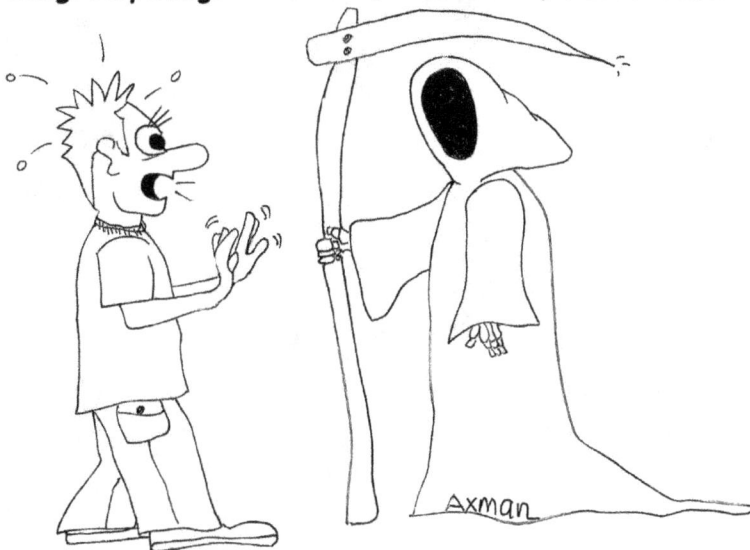

Your Mental Health Options

Remember the anxiety, depression, and anger that you felt (maybe) after the initial diagnosis? Even if you didn't have strong emotions then, you may experience strong emotions now. This time you may feel anger toward your doctor and anyone else who gave you recommendations. What were they thinking! The anger and depression can immobilize you. You might feel like giving up and doing nothing. That's a pretty common reaction at this time.

Don't let your emotions stop you from making a decision or taking further action. Get help for sure. Don't wait too long. You have a cancer that has already shown it has the ability to withstand treatment. Be sure you're the one in charge of deciding what your next course of action will be. You're the decider!

My Story

In spite of all the side effects, my strongest reaction was to yell yippee! I'm cured again, says I. Initially, my urologist/surgeon (Dr. W) told me the chance for surgical cure was about 95 percent and the radiation oncologist (Dr. N) said cure was 95 percent certain with the radiation. So now my overall chance of cure was a whopping 190 percent! Who could ask for more? I was guaranteed to be cured, and could give away another 90 percent to some other poor soul who really needed it!

I ran a marathon three months after radiation therapy, just to prove, again, I could do it. I went to another country where nobody would recognize me and only strangers would know how slow I was. I discovered that grumbling, complaining, and swearing were common to many languages. I barely made it through the 26.2 miles (42 km). I was pretty slow—about an hour slower than my previous slowest slow marathon. I experienced a multitude of pains and cramps and some major fatigue. I was still weak and tired from the radiation, and then there was that nasty rash on my backside.

In hindsight, it was probably not such a wise decision. I should have taken more time to recover and train. Better I should have stayed home and run one about six months later. But I did experience a feeling of accomplishment!

Please help me, I'm falling.

A couple months later, in celebration of my recovery and being alive and well on my 65th birthday, I jumped out of an airplane—solo. Yes, I actually had a parachute—and even a spare.

Floating down from 13,000 feet was a lot easier than running a marathon and very calming and relaxing. And I knew that sooner or later I'd get down to the ground; and I did.

So, once again, I had proven my inherent macho nature, such as it was. Even though I am a really tough guy, my recovery from radiation therapy took a lot (a lot) longer than I had anticipated. It actually took about a year—just like the doctor predicted—go figure. But this time I was finally cured once and for all! I'll drink to that! And I did.

8

Never Say Die—or Even Think It!

My Story

I've confirmed it yet again: Life really is not fair.

Another year has passed all too quickly (they all seem to pass quickly, he said philosophically). That undetectable PSA level shortly after the end of my final radiation treatment (the second treatment that was sure to cure me forever—remember?) has started increasing again—even faster than before. Unusual, says Dr. W. Seldom happens, says Dr. N. Somehow being unusual and unique in this situation doesn't make me feel all that special. And those incontinence and impotence issues from past treatments are gradually getting a little more noticable. When it rains it pours. And I live in Oregon where it always rains.

The choices narrow. After surgery and radiation, the remaining list of treatments that are likely to (or even just might) cure my prostate cancer has been reduced to about zero (nada). That doesn't mean there isn't treatment; there is just no realistic hope of cure at this time and stage of medical development. So it's back to square one for me.

I'll see more doctors, look for new treatments (clinical trials included), and try not to become discouraged, depressed, despondent, or a pain in the butt to my family and friends. Too late—I'm already a pain in the butt. I know prostate cancer generally grows slowly, and I believe that I'll probably stay alive long enough for some enterprising researcher to find a cure. It could happen. I'm thinking there's a pretty good chance it will happen.

And When Everything You Do Doesn't Work

You were treated for prostate cancer and it came back. Your secondary treatment didn't do the job, either. Your PSA is on the rise again.

Cancers that keep coming back can eventually become identified as incurable (that doesn't necessarily mean untreatable, remember?). Many men live many years with incurable prostate cancer. There are medications that have been and are being designed to slow prostate cancer growth in one way or another—some of them still in the testing stages. Most of these treatments will have some side effects. You'll want to get all the information you can. Many new and potentially helpful treatments are in the clinical trial stages. The key words here are potential and trials.

The types of treatment your doctors can recommend and make available to you will vary with the seriousness of your condition, rate of growth, availability of medications, and maybe other considerations. Some treatments slow cancer growth for months or years, and others are used to prolong life for weeks or months when the cancer is in the late stages.

New medications and treatments are being discovered, invented, uncovered, created, rediscovered, and tested on a very regular basis.

That's good. Sometimes a medication used for treating another cancer or even an unrelated disease shows promise for treating prostate cancer. If you have prostate cancer that has not responded to regular treatments, you probably wonder why research into new medications and cures is so slow. You want a cure now. In many areas of health, drugs have been discovered that result in medical cures, but it is often a very slow process taking years or decades to prove that they are safe and effective enough to gain FDA approval.

When Prostate Cancer Is Not Curable

Hormone or Androgen Deprivation Therapy is the most common treatment when prostate cancer is incurable—as discussed in chapter 4. Most men would rather not risk the side effects of ADT, but if it would help them to stay alive a while longer, it's worth consideration.

Androgen Deprivation Therapy can slow prostate cancer cell growth for several years. It has been effective in prolonging life when there are no more cures to try.

ADT Therapies Can Have Side Effects (doesn't everything have side effects?)

You may or may not have any of these side effects, but as the ADT suppresses the production of testosterone you may be at risk for some of these:

Anemia—the blood is less able to carry oxygen to body cells.

Cholesterol changes—cholesterol levels may increase due to weight gain.

Cognitive impairments—memory loss may occur.

Depression—feelings of sadness or disinterest may become stronger.

Edema—swelling in the legs due to water retention can develop.

Fatigue—feelings of being tired or having low energy are common.

Genital atrophy—the penis and scrotum may shrink.

Gynecomastia—the breasts may enlarge and become tender.

Hair changes—body hair may decrease and scalp hair may increase.

Erectile dysfunction/loss of libido—inability to achieve an erection or even feel sexual stimulation is possible.

Hot flashes—sudden feelings of warmth or heat may last for a few seconds or a few minutes and occur numerous times each day.

Muscle atrophy—loss of muscle mass and strength can occur.

Musculoskeletal pain—muscles and joints may become painful.

Osteoporosis or bone loss—bones can weaken and the risk of fracture can increase.

Thyroid problems—thyroid levels can go down.

Weight gain—non-muscle weight gain around the abdomen is common.

But living with side effects has its positive points. The most positive part is you're still alive. Pinch yourself to make sure. And you are unlikely to experience all or even most of these possible side effects.

My Story

More than a pair of docs.

Dr. W, the surgeon who referred me to Dr. N, the radiologist, now referred me to Dr. B, the oncologist and clinical trial expert. My health insurance provider and I are getting to know a lot of expensive doctors. In looking for clinical trials that might benefit me, I found that there are waiting lists for some trials and long waits for government approval for others.

So, in consultation with Dr. B, my new oncologist, I first volunteered to join a clinical trial and try an experimental drug. It didn't work for me or anybody else. No harm no foul.

Androgen Deprivation Therapy was the most common next step I was told. Women are well aware of the effects of estrogen. It is largely responsible for their feminine characteristics and ability to reproduce. I have no desire to become motherly, and then there's the hot flashes.

ADT, taken over a period of time, could cause changes in my shape (more hips, larger breasts— shapes I enjoy looking at, but not having) and pretty much eliminates the old sex drive (because of the side effects from previous treatments, this may not be much of a change). But ADT could slow my PSA increases for several years. That's good but I know it is not a cure.

So I entered the world of ADT. Over the past few years, I have used several types of ADT (pills and injections) which, for awhile slowed the increase of my PSA. That's a good outcome. The intense hot flashes were an added benefit.

Chemotherapy

When other treatments are no longer effective, particularly when Androgen Deprivation Therapy is no longer effective, chemotherapy is the most common next step. When hormones or hormone-like drugs no longer work, the condition is known as hormone refractory prostate cancer (HRPC).

You may take chemo once a day, once a week, once a month, or even less frequently. You may skip a month or more. How long you take chemo also depends on the type of cancer, how you respond to the drugs, and what length of time research has shown produces the best treatment results. Chemotherapy often helps reduce the pain associated with late-stage prostate cancer.

Various chemical cocktails have been created to try to slow prostate cancer growth when no other treatment works. At this time chemotherapy does not cure prostate cancer, but in some cases can add weeks or months to your survival.

Most chemotherapy drugs are taken in one of the following ways:

- It might be as easy as taking a pill or swallowing a liquid, and you can often do it at home, as long as you follow your doctor's directions.
- Chemo can be injected. The shots may be given in your doctor's office, a hospital, a clinic, or even at home.
- Most often, however, chemo is given right into your veins through a needle or tiny plastic tube. This is called an IV (intravenous) injection or drip.

Keep asking questions and checking the research. Because new chemical combinations are constantly being tried, there could be a breakthrough at any time.

Beware the Promises of Cure Online—for a price.

If you Google PROSTATE CANCER, you'll find tens of thousands of sites with information, suggestions, and the promise of useful treatments. You'll also find some sites that will guarantee cures for a price. But beware. If it sounds too good to be true... well, you know the rest. Always check things out with your medical team.

Natural, New, and Experimental Approaches

When none of the traditional therapies stops the relentless increase in PSA scores, you start looking for other things to try. There are a lot of products and procedures out there that claim to slow growth, stop growth, or even cure you. Many of these approaches fall under the title of CAM therapies—complementary and alternative therapies.

Just to set the record straight, at this time after radiation, surgery, cryosurgery, and other traditional treatments have been tried and have not been successful, there is no complementary or alternative treatment known that will cure prostate cancer. So you can pass right over the guaranteed cure possibilities. But there may be foods and other natural supplements and products that could help in slowing prostate cancer growth in some men. Proof is scarce. You may or may not want to try any of these approaches and your doctor may tell you they are useless or at least not proven. It's your choice.

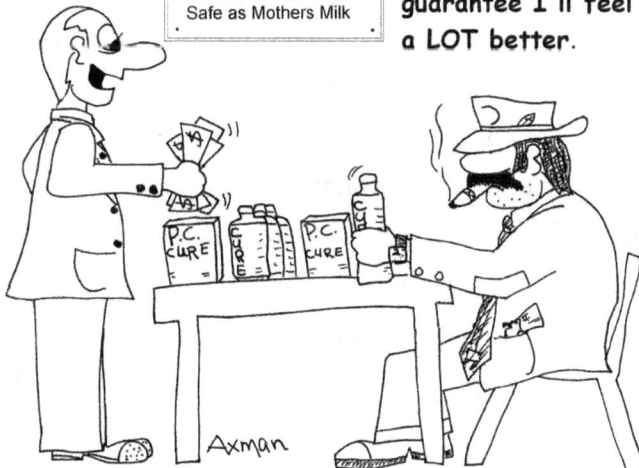

But just in case you're interested, here is a partial list of foods and supplements that have been shown to slow the growth of prostate cancer in some studies for some men (and more in mice).

Sometimes just in the lab and other times just in animals; most of these substances are not harmful to you and you may decide they're worth a try.

ANTIOXIDANTS

Antioxidants are substances in foods and supplements that may protect cells from the damage caused by unstable molecules known as free radicals. Free radical damage may lead to cancer. Antioxidants stabilize free radicals and may prevent some of the damage free radicals otherwise might cause. Antioxidants are available in many foods, and eating more fruits and vegetables seems like a no-brainer. The early promise of antioxidants as a way to prevent, cure, or slow cancer growth has not been shown to be as significant as first hoped. But dietary antioxidants might help make you healthier and are not known to be harmful in recommended amounts. Antioxidants have not been shown to cure existing cancer.

In recent years, large-scale, randomized clinical trials involving antioxidants have reached inconsistent and inconclusive results. That means that results are not proven, not that the substances don't help. And they may help one man and not another.

Want a technical explanation? Exposure to various environmental factors, including tobacco smoke and radiation, can also lead to free radical formation. In humans, the most common form of free radicals is oxygen. When an oxygen molecule (O2) becomes electrically charged or "radicalized," it tries to steal electrons from other molecules, causing damage to the DNA and other molecules. Over time, such damage may lead to diseases including cancer. Antioxidants are often described as "mopping up" free radicals, meaning they neutralize the electrical charge and prevent the free radical from taking electrons from and damaging other molecules. Now you know.

Antioxidants exist naturally in fruits and vegetables, as well as in other foods including nuts, grains, and some meats, poultry, and fish. The following list describes food sources of common antioxidants:

Beta-carotene is found in many foods that are orange in color, including sweet potatoes, carrots, cantaloupe, squash, apricots, pumpkin, and mangos. Some green leafy vegetables including collard greens, spinach, and kale are also rich in beta-carotene. There is little evidence that it prevents or slows the growth of prostate cancer.

Lutein, best known for its association with healthy eyes, is abundant in green, leafy vegetables such as collard greens, spinach, and kale. Studies have not consistently shown a relationship between lutein and reduced prostate cancer cell growth.

Flaxseed, rich in omega-3 fatty acids, may be effective in slowing prostate tumor growth. The flaxseed must be ground because the shell is indigestible. In a small study, 30 grams of ground flaxseed daily was shown to significantly slow tumor growth. Stay tuned for more results. Ground flaxseed is not the same as flaxseed oil.

Vitamin A is found in liver, sweet potatoes, carrots, milk, egg yolks, and mozzarella cheese. There is little evidence that it prevents or slows the growth of prostate cancer. High levels can be toxic.

Vitamin C is also called ascorbic acid and can be found in abundance in many fruits and vegetables and is also found in cereals, beef, poultry, and fish. There are ongoing studies to determine if vitamin C has a role in preventing or slowing prostate cancer.

Vitamin D, specifically, vitamin D3. The human body produces vitamin D3 when exposed to natural sunlight. So a little sunshine might help. This is a good and logical reason to visit someplace with a warm and sunny climate during the winter. Milk has high levels of vitamin D added. From 1000 to 1100 International Units (IU) of vitamin D3 daily has been shown to reduce overall cancer risk and inhibit (slow) prostate cancer growth in some, but not all, men with prostate cancer. Do not take high doses of vitamin D3 without medical approval and supervision. There is a blood test to determine whether you are deficient in vitamin D3. Most people are.

Vitamin E, also known as alpha-tocopherol, is found in almonds, in many oils including wheat germ, safflower, corn, and soybean oils, and is also found in mangos, nuts, broccoli, and other foods. It has long been thought to slow the growth of prostate cancer tumors. However, in a recent study, Vitamin E and Selenium wre found to have no protective effects against prostate cancer. Talk with your doctor before taking these supplements.

Lycopene. Studies of the prostate benefits of lycopene have been inconclusive. Many doctors recommend eating tomatoes (cooked, as tomato sauce, and even ketchup) as a possible protection against prostate cancer. Lycopene supplements are also available, but be sure to check with your doctor before taking a lycopene supplement.

OTHER OPTIONS

Capsaicin is the ingredient that makes hot peppers hot. Eating a jalapeno or habanera pepper can burn your mouth, tongue, and even your stomach. It also has been shown to help kill prostate cancer cells. It does this by causing cancer cells to age and die more like normal cells. Capsaicin has also been shown to cause tumors to shrink. It can be taken in pill form as well as by eating hot peppers and is available over the counter in cayenne capsules. Eating three to eight habanero peppers a week will meet the same level of capsaicin.

Jalapeno peppers also contain capsaicin, but at a lower level. Talk with your doctor about trying capsaicin.

Pomegranate juice. Research at UCLA found that men with recurrent prostate cancer who drank 8 ounces of pomegranate juice each day had cancer progression slowed by an average of 35 percent. Pomegranate juice is high in antioxidants, but it is not known for sure that this is the reason for the slower cancer cell growth. Whatever the reason, the results have been confirmed. Eight ounces of pomegranate juice a day slows PSA growth and increases the time before other treatments may become necessary.

Omega-3 fatty acids are found in fish oil and to lesser degrees in leafy green vegetables, nuts, sesame seeds, and some vegetable oils. Research has shown that increasing omega-3 fatty acids and reducing omega-6 fatty acids (found in corn oil, flaxseed oil, and other vegetable sources) can slow the growth of prostate cancer cells. Normally, Americans eat omega-6 and omega-3 fatty acids in a 15-1 ratio (15 times more omega-6). The recommended ratio for slowing cancer growth is 1 to 1.

ABM mushrooms. The ABM mushroom Agaricus originated in a small area of Brazil. It has been used for alternative cancer treatment for more than 30 years. There is very little evidence of its effect on slowing prostate cancer cell growth at this time, however. Always check with your doctor before trying an unknown substance.

Green tea. Japanese and Chinese men who regularly drink green tea have a lower risk of prostate cancer than their peers who did not drink green tea and most other ethnic groups. Clinical studies have shown mixed results. It may or may not help slow prostate cancer growth, but probably does no harm and may help in other ways.

Black tea. Recent studies have shown that black tea slows prostate cancer cell growth in men with advanced prostate cancer. Men in the studies drank up to five cups of black tea each day.

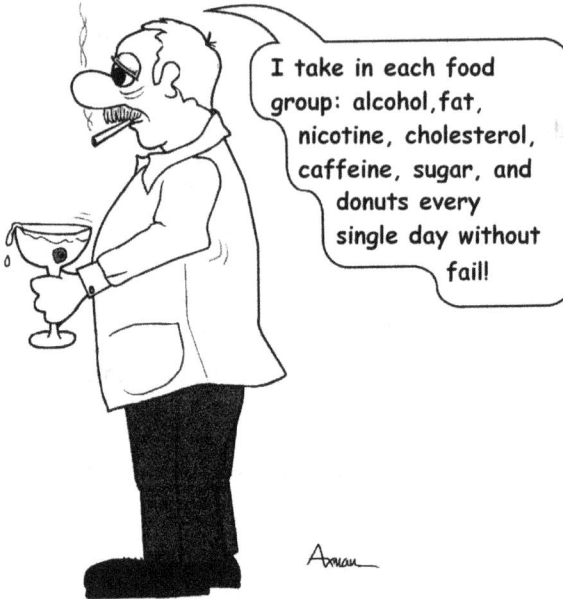

Soy protein. Soy products, such as tofu, contain phytoestrogens, which are compounds that have estrogen-like activity. Estrogen, and drugs that act like estrogen, is used to treat late-stage prostate cancer by reducing the effects of testosterone on prostate cancer cell growth. In cultures where soy products are commonly eaten, the incidence of prostate cancer is lower than in other cultures. Studies are under way to determine the exact mechanisms involved.

Macrobiotic Diet

The basic macrobiotic diet consists of five categories of foods (with recommended weight percentage of total food consumed):

- Whole grains (40%-60%), including brown rice, barley, millet, oats, wheat, corn, rye, and buckwheat; and other less common grains and products made from them, such as noodles, bread, and pasta.

- Vegetables (20%-30%), including small amounts of raw or pickled vegetables—preferably locally grown and prepared in a variety of ways.
- Beans (5%-10%), such as azuki, chickpeas, or lentils; other bean products, such as tofu, tempeh, or natto.
- Regular consumption of sea vegetables, such as nori, wakame, kombu, and hiziki—cooked either with beans or as separate dishes.
- Foods such as fruit, white fish, seeds, and nuts—to be consumed a few times per week or less often.

The standard macrobiotic diet avoids foods that include meat and poultry, animal fats (such as lard and butter), eggs, dairy products, refined sugar, and foods containing artificial sweeteners or other chemical additives.

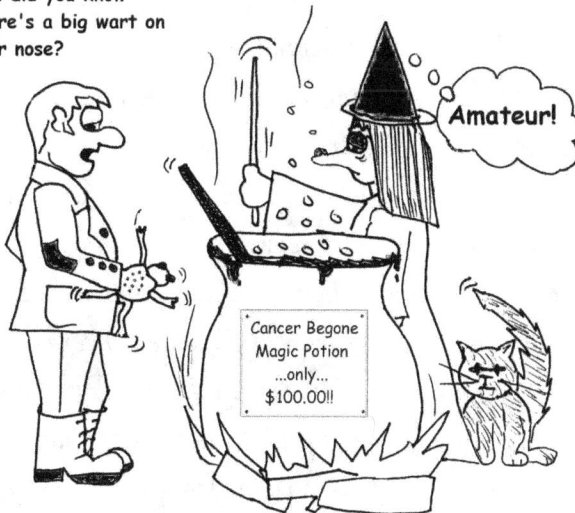

Some men with advanced prostate cancer believe they have slowed or stopped cancer growth by adhering to a macrobiotic diet. It may be a difficult diet to maintain and the evidence of success is mixed.

My Story

Smoke and mirrors. Those out-of-the-ordinary approaches.

By talking with doctors, searching the Internet (and sorting the wheat from the chaff from the herbs), talking to friends, and reading medical journal articles (no easy task), I found several articles and results from studies that suggested simple, inexpensive, and natural things I could do that might, maybe, possibly slow down my cancer growth (note: no more talk of cure). In many cases the results were based on testing with mice and rats, but how different could they be? And I've already been called a rat a time or two.

My diet has changed a little. Natural approaches are certainly worth a try for me—little risk and maybe even some good results. There is not much information about the results of using several of the complementary approaches at the same time— so I drink pomegranate juice a few times a week, eat hot peppers a couple times a week, and take vitamin D3 supplements every day. I drink a cup of green tea whenever I remember. Each of these supplements has been shown to kill or slow growth in prostate cancer cells in some studies. And no studies I have seen show negative side effects.

Vitamin E used to be considered helpful but has fallen from favor—at least this week—so I don't take any. The information and recommendations keep changing. So far there have been no problems with the interactions of any of these substances, but one never knows. I'm not suggesting that you or anyone else should try this—remember the "Don't try this at home" admonition. But, after a few months of pomegranate juice and hot peppers, my PSA rate of increase actually slowed down a little. Something was helping—it could just be the clean living and pure thoughts. But of course, it didn't last

VITAMINS IN MODERATION

A recent study from the National Cancer Institute found that taking larger-than-recommended doses of vitamins (more than one multivitamin a day) could increase the risk for advanced and fatal prostate cancer in men already diagnosed with prostate cancer. Taking one daily multivitamin had no negative effect, but men who took high doses of vitamins were at increased risk.

A University of Michigan urologist suggests that men with prostate cancer take a daily multivitamin, but it must be a formulation for postmenopausal women. These multis contain no iron (you don't need iron) but do contain plenty of needed calcium and vitamin D3. Ask your doctor if you need any supplements.

Clinical Trials (and Tribulations)

By now just about everybody has heard the term clinical trial. In the realm of prostate cancer, numerous drugs or treatments are being tested for effectiveness. Volunteers are recruited by doctors, clinics, or even online—these new approaches or medications haven't been totally proven or yet approved by the FDA. Some trials are for men at early stages of cancer; others for men near the end of the cycle.

If you have recently been diagnosed with cancer, if your cancer has returned, or if it is not responding to treatment, you may be a good candidate for a clinical trial. How do you know? First, talk to your doctor.

CLINICAL TRIALS CENTER

Here's the new trial drug! It has eye of newt, toe of frog, wing of bat, and tongue of dog! Wow!!

I think I've heard of this formula before...

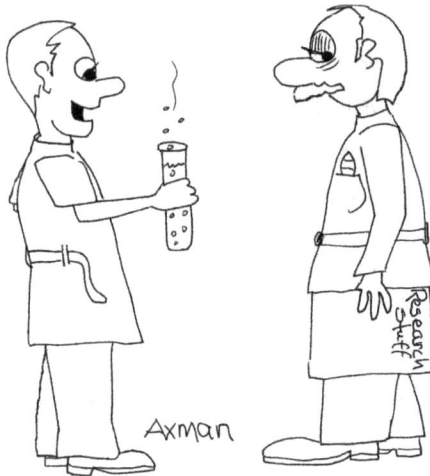

Axman

What Is a Clinical Trial?

Clinical trials are people-based studies—as opposed to studies done in laboratories with mice and other animals or in test tubes—of new drugs or procedures. Doctors and researchers use clinical trials to learn whether a new treatment is safe and effective in patients. Such studies are necessary in the development of new treatments for many serious diseases including prostate cancer. No medication is approved by the FDA unless it has been successfully tested in clinical trials.

The doctors and researchers in charge of a clinical trial don't know ahead of time exactly how things will turn out. If they did, there would be no need for the study in the first place. Because of this, there's no simple answer to the question, "Should I take part and what are the risks?" Your participation could help you and advance the knowledge and treatment. Or it could cause damage—but the chances of a negative result are low because the ingredients and dosages have already undergone preliminary testing leading up to the clinical trial approval.

Sometimes a clinical trial will test one group getting the standard treatment (let's say, drugs A and B) against another group of similar patients who also get the standard treatment plus the "trial drug" (drugs A and B and C).

My Story

*Knowing I have an incurable disease is not very comforting. I seldom even think the word **terminal**. Of course, life itself is terminal and everybody has to die of something, sometime, he said bravely. Knowing that eventually the cancer could kill me is rather grim, but I still prefer knowing to not knowing. I have never believed that ignorance was bliss—except in politics and how sausages are made. And thinking the worst and worrying about what might happen next doesn't serve any useful purpose—it might even make things worse. Not that I don't think and worry a little, but I try not to dwell on my own tribulations and rather focus on living the best I can for as long as I can. Keep busy, keep active, and keep on keeping on. I walk, write, run, draw cartoons, read, travel, and find reasons to laugh (mostly at myself just like everybody else does).*

Keeping the cancer slowed down may give that enterprising

scientist somewhere (are you listening young—or even old—researcher?) a little more time to find a cure or treatment that will slow down cell growth for years and years and years. I think it could happen. I'm waiting.

Most people don't pay much attention to clinical trials until they are diagnosed with a serious illness such as prostate cancer and run out of traditional treatment options. Medical breakthroughs (the results of clinical trials) may sometimes make the evening news, but you usually don't hear about clinical trials themselves unless something has gone wrong. The media are quick to pick up on an instance when a volunteer in a study is harmed. While it is very rare, people have been harmed and have even died while taking part in clinical trials. Reports of these tragic outcomes are important, because they help to expose problems in the system, which are then corrected to protect others.

What you don't usually hear about, however, are the thousands of brave people who are helped each year because they decided to take part in a clinical trial, not to mention the millions who ultimately benefit from the participation of others. Help is usually in the form of extended life or improved quality of life, but not cure—so far.

There is no right or wrong choice when it comes time for you to decide whether or not to take part in a clinical trial. The decision is a very personal one and depends on many factors, including the potential benefits and risks of the study and what you hope to achieve by taking part.

Knowing all you can about clinical trials in general—and ones you are considering in particular—can help you feel more at ease with your decision. When you're considering whether or not to participate, knowing what to look for and what to expect can help you make a wiser decision.

What are the benefits of participating in a clinical trial (if any)?

- You may be cured for minimal cost. That's a great (but rare) outcome. It sometimes happens (but not yet with prostate cancer).
- You may not be cured, but the cancer growth rate may be slowed. This is a more likely outcome. It happens with some trials. But there may also be side effects that can cause concern.
- Nothing may happen. You may see no improvement but also no worsening of your condition.
- There may be adverse effects. There may be problems with your heart, liver, blood pressure, or something else. When this happens, the trials are usually stopped. In any clinical trial, you can choose to stop participating at any time.

The final choice is always up to you, but take a serious look at available trials. Very few people participate in clinical trials and some potentially helpful drugs are never tested.

My Story

I'm off to the next level—whatever it may bring. It all sounds kind of adventurous. Anything that might help is worth looking at. Guys with incurable prostate cancer often live a long time and die from something else (this may actually be more encouraging than it sounds). Or, to quote Dr. W, "You'll probably get hit by a bus long before the cancer kills you."

Participating in a Clinical Trial

First, talk with your doctor or medical care team. They often know about trials or can refer you to someone or someplace where there is credible information (check out chapter 10). Don't rush into any trial. Different trials may be available in different locations. Are you prepared to travel across the state or country to find the one you want? Some men do. But a network of cancer doctors throughout the country, coordinated by the National Cancer Institute, can offer you state-of-the-art cancer treatment through trials at many medical centers (perhaps one near you).

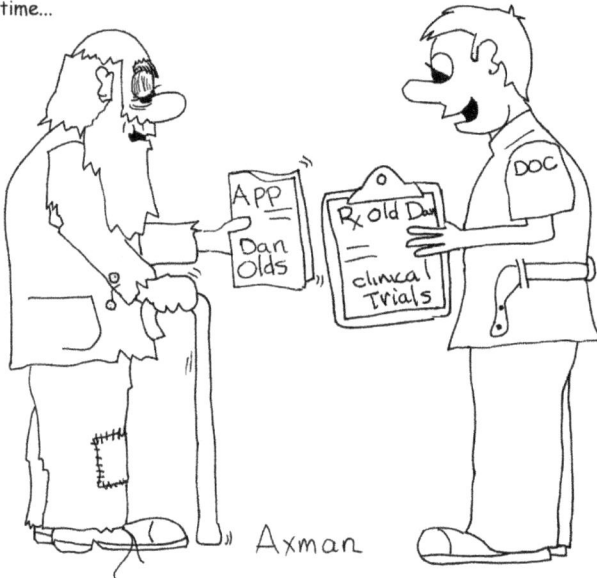

What you need to know BEFORE becoming a participant:
- What is the purpose of the study?
- Does it fit with your purposes?
- Does it deal specifically with prostate cancer treatment at your stage and grade?

- What kinds of tests and treatment are involved?
- What does this treatment do or what is it supposed to do?
- What is likely to happen to me, with or without this treatment?
- What are my other choices?
- What are the advantages and disadvantages?
- How could participation affect my daily life?
- What side effects can I expect? Can these side effects be managed?
- Will I have to be hospitalized? If so, how often and for how long?
- Will any or all of the treatment be free?
- Will my health insurance cover any of the costs? Often insurance companies pay for standard treatment, and the drug company pays for the experimental medication. Medicare pays for standard treatment if you are over 65, and most states require health insurance providers to do the same.
- Could I be harmed as a result of participating?
- Would I be treated for any side effects?
- What type of long-term follow-up care does the study provide?
- Has the treatment been used to treat other diseases or types of cancers? With what results?
- How long will the trial last?
- Are there other, more promising, clinical trials available or on the horizon for which I might qualify?

Be sure you get the answers you want and feel comfortable with the whole process before you agree to participate. Remember, the hospitals, doctors, and drug companies want the trials to work.

There are three phases of clinical trials in which a treatment is studied before it is eligible for approval by the FDA (Food and Drug

Administration).

Phase I clinical trials: The purpose of a phase I study is to find the best way to administer a new treatment by pills, injection, or liquid, and how much of it can be given safely. The cancer care team watches patients carefully for any harmful side effects. The treatment has already been tested in lab and animal studies, but the side effects in patients are not completely known. Doctors conducting the clinical trial often start by giving very low doses of the drug to the first patients and increasing the dose for later groups of patients until side effects appear. Although doctors are hoping to help patients, the main purpose of a phase I study is to test the safety of the drug. The number of participants is usually low.

Phase II clinical trials: These studies are designed to see if the drug actually works (benefits outweigh risks and side effects). Participants are usually given the highest dose that doesn't cause adverse side effects (determined from the phase I study) and closely observed for an effect on the cancer. The cancer care team also looks for previously unknown side effects. Participants are asked to keep careful records and report any and all side effects or unusual responses to the experimental drug or procedure. Participants are closely monitored. The length of phase II studies can vary from several months to several years.

Phase III clinical trials: Phase III studies involve large numbers of participants—often several hundred or thousands. In a typical phase III procedure, one group (the control group) receives the current gold standard (most accepted treatment—if there is one) and another group receives the new treatment. All patients in Phase III studies are closely watched. The study will be stopped if the side effects of the new treatment are too severe or if one group has had much better results than the other. If the treatment proves to be safe and effective, FDA approval and general availability of the drug will follow.

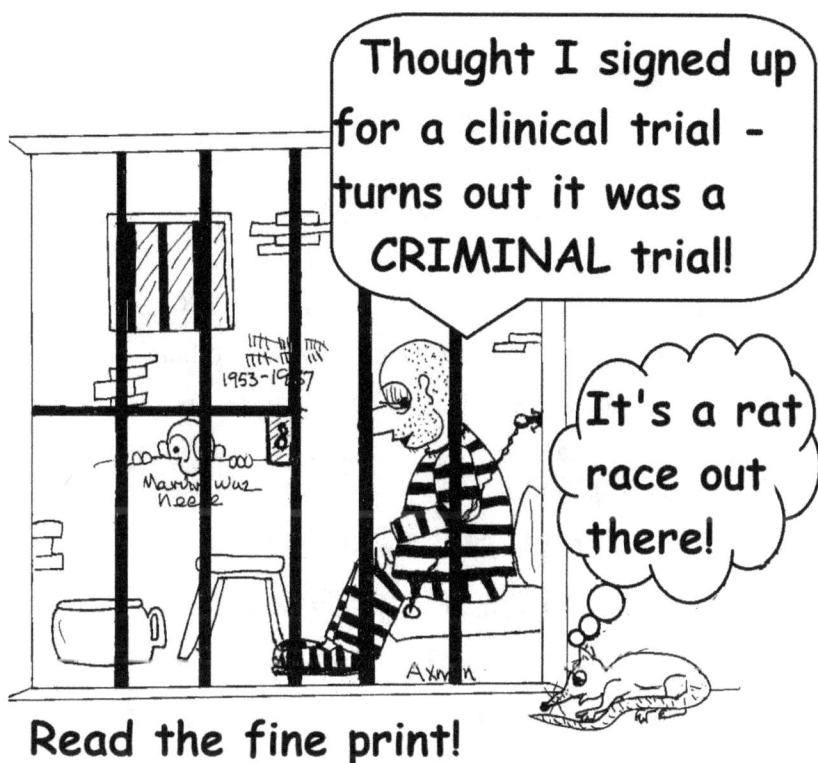

Read the fine print!

A New Direction in Medications

In the last several years, a number of new medications have been tested that use the individual's immune system as the cancer fighting agent. One of these new vaccines has already been approved by the FDA and is in use to extend lives in some men with late stage prostate cancer. It is called Provenge® (sipuleucel-T).

This vaccine uses the individual patient's immune cells to help identify and attack prostate cancer cells. The success of personalized vaccines may change the way prostate cancer is treated in the future.

Numerous other promising prostate cancer drugs are being tested and may be available to by the time you're reading this. Check with your oncologist about these new drugs and clinical trials that might benefit you. As drugs are approved for late-stage treatment, some of them are being tested in clinical trials on men with earlier stages of prostate cancer.

MDV3100 (it will have a more sophisticated name when it is approved by the FDA...if it is approved) is in phase III studies as this is written. And watch for drugs with names like Yervoy, Cabozantinib, and Zytiga down the line. There certainly will be others.

You can bet that one reality of using any new drugs will be a high cost. Having good health insurance can be very important.

Final Stage Decisions

Sometimes all the treatments you try don't stop the cancer and it continues to grow. You may get sick, weak, and eventually must face death. You may be afraid and feel alone even if you have a loving family and a good support group.

Supporting Someone with Late-Stage Cancer

What do you say to a person who is dying or talks about dying? This is something that happens to people every day, but may have never happened to anyone you know. Everybody handles it in a different way. Some will want to know all the details—just how and when they will die. What will actually happen in the dying process? For answers to this question, you will need to seek experts in hospice care or care of the terminally ill. They can guide you in understanding just what might happen—if you really want to know.

Hospice staff are trained in answering those questions every day, and they are skilled in providing useful and accurate information in a supportive way. In many communities, hospice organizations provide expert and compassionate care for people with a variety of advanced and terminal diseases.

If someone close to you is dying, you don't have to know all the answers—just be there and be supportive. Let the person cry or talk about their life, good times, experiences, sadness, and regrets— if they choose to. You can be a good listener often without having to respond at all. Allowing a person to talk can be helpful to them. Many people are very uncomfortable with any talk of death and won't allow themselves to feel the pain with a friend or loved one. That's their choice; it doesn't have to be yours.

Some men will feel more comfortable getting support and counseling from a spiritual advisor.

Advance Directives

Everyone has the right to make some decisions about his or her own health care. This includes deciding when and if you want medical treatment to continue or to stop. You have the right to accept or refuse treatments, even treatments that might prolong your life. One way to hold onto your rights is by putting decisions about future health care in writing. This is called an advance directive or living will. An advance directive is a legal paper. It can state your wishes about health care choices. Or it can name someone else to make those choices if you cannot. Doctors, in most cases, must follow your advance directive if you can't make medical decisions because of an illness or injury.

Advance directives can only be used for decisions about medical care. The exact form of an advance directive varies from state to state or from one country to another. A senior center, hospice program, your doctor, or a lawyer can help you get the right form, fill it out, and have it witnessed. If you have a serious disease or are just getting older, it could be wise to draw up an advance directive while your mind is sound and before a difficult medical situation should arise.

9

That Other Manly Cancer

Just in case you want another cancer to worry about, there's an additional all-male cancer you should know. It's called testicular cancer, but it might be better known to you as Lance Armstrong's disease. The good news is—he survived it and went on to win fame and fortune.

If you're old enough to be concerned about prostate cancer, you're probably too old to worry much about testicular cancer. But you probably have sons or grandsons who are at an age when testicular cancer is a concern.

Testicular cancer is mostly a problem for young men. If you're middle-aged or older, warn your sons, grandsons, nephews, and other young men you may know. Young men often feel invincible and don't see much risk—they're in their prime—young, strong, and energetic. Cancer is the farthest thing from their mind. But now is when they should be checking themselves regularly for testicular cancer.

Testicles produce, store, and secrete sperm, and are also the body's main source of male hormones. The hormones are responsible for your masculine characteristics such as low voice and body hair and they also control the development of your reproductive organs.

Each year about 10,000 American men are diagnosed with cancer of the testicles, which accounts for only about 1 percent of all cancers in men. Those statistics make it sound rare. However, in men aged 20 to 34, testicular cancer is the most commonly diagnosed cancer. It's only later on that they'll be focused mostly on prostate cancer.

Risk Factors

No one knows for sure what causes cancer to form in the testicles. But a few risk factors are known:

- **Age:** Testicular cancer is the most common cancer in men between the ages of 20 to 34, the second most common cancer in men 35 to 39, and the third most common cancer between the ages of 15 to 19.
- **Race:** Testicular cancer is more common among white men than black men. Hispanic, American Indian, and Asian men develop testicular cancer at a higher rate than black men, but lower than white men.
- **Family history:** Men with a family history of testicular cancer (and even breast cancer) may have an increased risk of the disease.

Hereditary Conditions

- **Gonadal dysgenesis:** A rare genetic disorder in females that inhibits normal sexual development and causes infertility. If a man's female relatives have/had it, he is at increased risk for testicular cancer.
- **Klinefelter's syndrome:** Low levels of male hormones, sterility, breast enlargement, and small testes characterize this sex chromosome disorder.

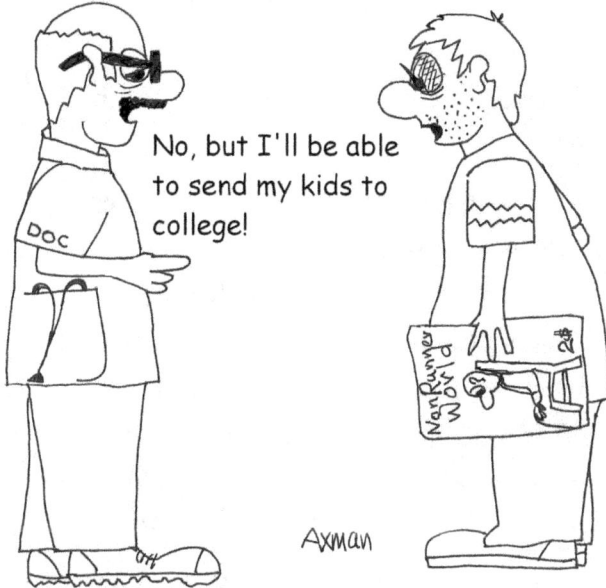

I prescribe more X-rays, blood texts, scans, injections and drugs.

Will I be cured then, Doc, huh? Will I?

No, but I'll be able to send my kids to college!

DOC

NonRunner World

Axman

Personal History

- **Testicular cancer:** If you've had testicular cancer in one testicle before, you're at increased risk of developing cancer in your other testicle.

- **Undescended testicle:** Normally the testicles descend into the scrotum before birth. Even if surgery is performed to place the testicle in the scrotum, the risk of testicular cancer is increased.

- **Abnormal testicular development:** Men whose testicles did not develop normally are at increased risk.

According to the National Cancer Institute, there is practically no association between vasectomy (sterilization by having the vas deferens tubes adjacent to the testicles cut) and testicular cancer (or prostate cancer).

Symptoms

Men themselves discover most testicular cancers—either by accident or while performing self-examination. Your doctor should also examine your testicles for any abnormality as part of your routine physical. If you find anything unusual about your testicles, contact your doctor right away:

- A painless lump or swelling in either testicle
- Any enlargement of a testicle
- Any change in the way your testicle feels
- A feeling of heaviness in the scrotum
- A dull ache in your lower abdomen or groin
- A sudden collection of fluid in the scrotum
- Pain or discomfort in a testicle or in the scrotum

These symptoms could be caused by conditions other than cancer, so your doctor will need to examine you to know for sure—and possibly order blood tests and other diagnostics. Cancer of the testicle is often completely curable when diagnosed and treated in the early stages.

10

Tell Me More, Tell Me More! Seeking Words of Wisdom

Always ask your doctor about any treatment, studies, or anything else you want to know. It's the right place to start. You can read the medical journals to focus on the latest research—it helps to have someone with a medical background explain all the long technical terms.

There is also a lot of prostate cancer information available in print and on the Internet. Some of it is accurate and helpful; some is not. It's not always easy to tell which is which. Always check and double-check your sources. When a piece of information tells you something that sounds too good to be true, the alarms should go off in your head. Some information may help SOME men and not others. Remember to always check out new information with your doctor.

There are literally thousands of information sites available on the Internet. Here are a few to help you get started.

Internet Links and Sources

Information is always changing. Even the site links may change but you can usually find what you want by putting the actual name of the site or organization into a search engine. You have the ability to get information for yourself and some would even say you owe it to yourself and your family to be as well informed as possible. The sites you visit should provide information telling you when the sites were last updated.

National Cancer Institute

www.cancer.gov/cancertopics

The NCI provides a wide variety of credible information, links, and recommendations. It is easy to navigate and easy to understand. The information is regularly updated. Look for clinical trials here. A good place to start searching.

American Cancer Society

www.cancer.org

The ACS provides accurate information and resources about all kinds of cancer, including prostate. There are links to additional information. The ACS site provides a large volume of up-to-date information. It's easy to find, easy to read, and accurate. This is a good one.

Malecare Prostate Cancer Support

www.malecare.org

Malecare is a national all-volunteer nonprofit organization providing a multilingual Web site with timely news as well as doctor- and patient-authored articles on prostate cancer. Malecare also offers in-person and online support groups, including a special group and articles specifically for gay men with prostate cancer. You can email questions and get answers from experts. Malecare has a BLOG site where information and discussion is available for men with advanced prostate cancer:
www.advancedprostatecancer.net.

Medline Plus—Prostate Cancer

www.nlm.nih.gov/medlineplus/prostatecancer.html
This government site provides medical and research information about prostate cancer. It is designed for health professionals, but just about anybody can find accurate cancer information. You may have to look up some of the medical terminology used. The results of the most recent research studies are available here.

Prostate Cancer Foundation

www.pcf.org
The Prostate Cancer Foundation raises money and funds high-impact research to find better treatments and a cure for prostate cancer. The site also provides news and research results. Check out their latest postings.

Prostate Cancer Research Institute

www.prostate-cancer.org
PCRI helpline: 1-800-641-7274. Be sure to have your own diagnostic and personal information ready when you call. PCRI is a nonprofit organization dedicated to assisting those with prostate cancer find educational materials, treatment options, updates on what side effects to expect, and information about various types of testing. It also publishes a quarterly newsletter.

US®TOO! International, Inc.

800-80-US TOO (800-808-7866)

www.ustoo.org
US TOO is a nonprofit organization that provides support and education for men with prostate cancer. The organization offers contact with support groups and provides the latest information about treatment for this disease.

Information About Clinical Trials

There are numerous clinical trials in progress all the time. Some are localized to a specific hospital or region and others are available nationwide or even worldwide. They vary in what their goals are, what kind of medical treatment you will receive, if any, and how long they last. Your first source of clinical trial information is your oncologist and medical team. You can also find information online. Discuss any information you find with your doctor to help determine if a clinical trial might be available and beneficial to you.

National Cancer Institute

www.cancer.gov/clinicaltrials/search/
NCI has a listing and search program where you can find clinical trials for your type and stage of cancer, in locations you choose, and links to those conducting the trials. When you find a possible trial, or have a question, check with your oncologist. NCI has a comprehensive database.

CancerNet

www.cancernet.nci.nih.gov/
This government Web site includes the PDQ—an NCI database that contains the latest information about cancer treatment, screening, prevention, genetics, supportive care, and complementary and alternative medicine, plus clinical trials with Cancer Trials searchable databases. The NCI's PDQ provides complete listings of NIH/NCI government-sponsored trials but not pharmaceutical/ proprietary industry trials. The following sites include clinical trial listings:

Center Watch

www.centerwatch.com

This site lists more than 40,000 government- and industry-sponsored clinical trials. You can search those trials that focus on prostate cancer. There are almost always listings of trials with available slots. When you find a possible trial, or have a question, check first with your oncologist.

Emergingmed.com

www.emergingmed.com

EmergingMed.com is a free and confidential cancer clinical trial matching and referral service. When you find a possible trial, or have a question, check first with your oncologist.

Acurian

www.acurian.com

The Acurian site will notify you when a trial becomes available that meets your reported needs. When you find a possible trial, or have a question, check first with your oncologist.

My Story

I am not dead yet!

Millions of people wake up every day knowing that they have an incurable or possibly fatal disease. You may be one of them. I'm one of them. It seems kind of melodramatic to say that. Sometimes I think briefly about that, but most of the time it's the furthest thing from my mind. As long as I'm busy and focused on what I'm doing, the details of mortality will just have to take care of themselves—as if there was another choice. I try to retain my gallows sense of humor—it amuses me even if those around me see it as a little bit morbid.

The system isn't perfect—yet. As I have gone through the processes, procedures, red tape, fights with health insurance providers, and problems scheduling appointments with doctors, labs, and hospitals, there have been some frustrations and discouraging moments. But I have done it all (as you probably would, too) because I'm concerned with my own treatment and survival.

In some medical situations it felt like I was just a number—a research subject (patient #45693- ax). Some doctors didn't remember who I was from one appointment to the next. In several cases I have had to drive long distances two days in a row because somebody did the wrong blood tests or the wrong tests were ordered or the right tests were NOT ordered. Medications have been unavailable when needed, personnel changes at clinics and hospitals have slowed the process, and sometimes I have had difficulty finding out the results of all those tests and procedures.

But, in most cases, being persistent and moderately patient (remember the part about me not being very patient?), and *smiling has ultimately resulted in getting almost everything done that needed to be done. **I have also met some great people—doctors, nurses, and fellow patients. That has been the best part.***

The Prostate Cancer Words

Let's talk Doc Talk. What it really means (probably) when your doctor or a journal article uses words like these:

Ablation—The removal of diseased or unwanted tissue from the body by surgery or other means.

Active Surveillance—Monitoring slow-growing prostate cancer through regular checkups rather than immediately treating it. Also called Watchful Waiting.

Adenocarcinoma—A cancer that begins in the cells lining and ducts and tubes of the prostate gland.

Androgen—A type of hormone that promotes the development and maintenance of male sex characteristics.

Anesthesia—The loss of sensation in any part of the body by the use of a numbing or paralyzing agent. Often used during surgery to put a person to sleep and keep them asleep during the procedure.

Androgen Deprivation Therapy (ADT)—Estrogen (a female hormone), or more likely drugs that act much like estrogen, is given to men to stop the testicles from producing testosterone. Testosterone helps prostate cancer cells grow and reproduce.

Bladder—The balloon shaped organ, a thin, flexible muscle that holds urine temporarily before being discharged through the urethra.

Benign—Not malignant; not cancerous.

Biopsy—A sampling of cells removed from the prostate by using a hollow needle inserted through the anus. The cells are examined under a microscope by experts to see if they are cancerous.

Bone scan—A test that detects areas of increased or decreased bone metabolism. The test is used to identify abnormal processes involving the bones such as tumors, infections, or fractures.

Brachytherapy—Also called internal radiation therapy, where small radioactive seeds are placed directly into the tumor.

Catheter—A thin tube that is inserted through the penis and urethra into the bladder to allow urine to drain or for performing certain procedures or tests.

Chemotherapy—Using drugs that will kill or slow the growth of cancer cells, usually after Androgen Deprivation Therapy has failed.

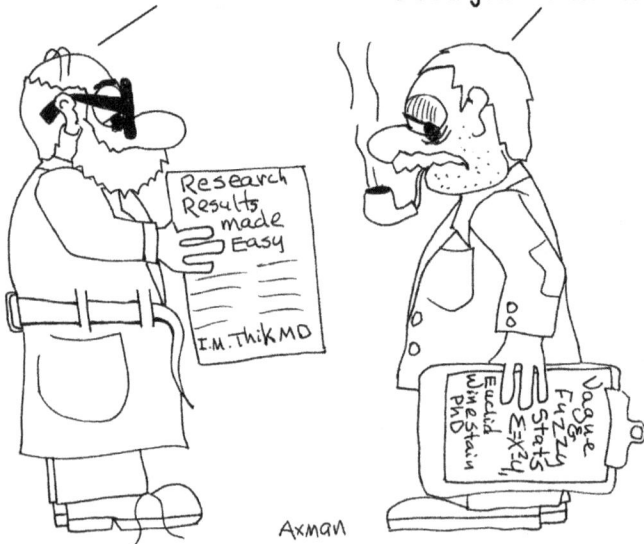

Clinical trial—New medications and treatments need to be tested on people with the disease being studied. This testing is done under close medical supervision, usually with volunteer participants.

Computed tomographic scan (CT scan)—A "CAT" scan is a type of x-ray that produces images of cross sections of the body. CT scans are more detailed than regular x-rays.

Conformal proton beam radiation therapy—Similar to external beam radiation therapy but uses proton beams instead of radiation to kill the cancer.

Cryosurgery—The freezing of a prostate tumor to destroy it and kill cancer cells.

Cyst—An abnormal growth or sac containing gas, fluid, or a semisolid material. Cysts may form in many parts of the body.

Cystoscope—A narrow, tubelike instrument fitted with lenses and a light that is passed through the urethra to look inside the bladder.

Digital rectal examination (DRE)—In this common prostate exam the doctor inserts a gloved, lubricated finger into the rectum to feel the prostate for swelling or abnormalities.

Erectile dysfunction (ED)—Also called impotence, it is the condition in men where they cannot achieve or maintain an erection.

External beam radiation therapy (EBRT)—This common prostate cancer treatment uses x-rays from an outside source, focused on the prostate gland, or the area where it was removed, to kill cancer cells.

Gleason Score—This system of grading the size and risk of a tumor by observing the characteristics of the cancerous cells in the tumor. Cell samples are taken through a biopsy.

Hormone—A natural chemical produced in the body and released into the blood to trigger or regulate functions of the body.

Hormonal therapy—Also known as androgen deprivation therapy. Estrogen (a female hormone), or drugs that act much like estrogen, is given to men to stop the testicles from producing testosterone.

IAD (intermittent androgen deprivation)—Using hormone therapy intermittently as a means to manage prostate cancer.

Impotence—Also called erectile dysfunction (ED), it is the condition in men where they cannot achieve or maintain an erection.

Incontinence—The inability to control urination. It can be (and often is) a side effect of prostate cancer treatment.

Indolent prostate cancer—This kind of prostate cancer is so slow growing that it rarely becomes a serious threat to health.

Intensity modulated radiation therapy (IMRT)— Similar to external beam radiation therapy, the machine delivering the radiation dose moves around the patient permitting radiation of varying intensity to be beamed from several directions.

Internal radiation therapy (also called brachytherapy)—Where small radioactive seeds are placed directly into the tumor.

Laparoscopic radical prostatectomy (LRP)—The prostate is removed using instruments inserted through small incisions and monitored through an optical device called a laparoscope.

My Story

Here I am, nine years down the road from that 2003 diagnosis. I have used a variety of meds—hormone treatments in recent years—and participated in three clinical trials. None of the trials cured me, stopped my cancer, or even slowed it down. But I definitely benefitted from the process. I have met some great people and am part of a very good support group as a result of one of the trials. I've learned a lot and hopefully that will help me in my future survival pursuits. Who said, "Old dogs can't learn new tricks?" I can't remember, of course, but he was dead wrong.

Could this whole process have worked out better? Probably. Should I back off and just wait to see what happens? Probably not. I have tried to keep my cool, roll with the punches, complain quietly (but firmly), and continue to do what I believe to be in my best interest (regardless of what may be in the best interest of the doctors, nurses, research studies, labs, and drug companies). In other words, I don't intend to give up. That may or may not, of course, make an iota of difference.

I continue to believe that some new treatment or new application of an old one is going to make a big difference one of these days. Probably everybody with any disease, condition, or problem thinks the same way—sometimes. I also believe that:

What is, is. What can go wrong, will. Life isn't for sissies. Nobody gets out of here alive.

(Add your own real life cliché in this space— it might be inspiring to some, amuse others, and failing all else it might make a fitting epitaph.)

Latent prostate cancer—The prostate cancer exists but produces no symptoms.

Luteinizing hormone releasing hormone (LHRH) analog—In this common form of hormone therapy, drugs block production of testosterone to slow the growth of prostate cancer cells or shrink the prostate tumor.

Lymph nodes—Small rounded masses of tissue distributed along the lymphatic system throughout the body. Lymph nodes produce cells that fight off foreign agents invading the body and trap infectious agents.

Lymphedema—The painful swelling of the lymph nodes in the body that may occur if the lymph nodes around the prostate are removed.

Metastasis—The spreading of cancer from one part of the body to another, such as from the prostate to the bones.

MRI (magnetic resonance imaging)—A diagnostic procedure using a combination of large magnets, radio frequencies, and a computer to produce detailed images of organs and structures within the body.

Oncologist—A doctor who specializes in cancer diagnosis and treatment.

Orchiectomy—This form of hormone therapy is accomplished by the surgical removal of the testes.

Penile prostheses—A semi-rigid or inflated device that is implanted into the penis to partially alleviate impotence.

Prostate gland—The walnut-sized organ in the male reproductive system located just below the bladder that produces a component of semen.

Prostate-specific antigen (PSA) test—PSA is a protein produced by the cells of the prostate gland. The PSA blood test measures the level of PSA in the blood. The higher the level of PSA, the greater the risk of prostate cancer.

Prostatitis—The prostate gland becomes infected. It is common, often painful, but treatable.

Radical prostatectomy—The surgical removal of the prostate gland.

Radiation therapy—The use of x-rays or other radiation sources, external or internal, to slow the growth of or kill cancer cells.

Radiotherapy—Another name for radiation therapy.

Resection—The surgical removal of a portion of a body part. When the prostate is removed, the urethra is severed in two places (resectioned) and must be reattached in order to function normally again.

Robotic prostate surgery—Robotic arms controlled externally by a doctor. Small incisions and reduced bleeding are characteristics of this surgical approach.

Seminal vesicles—Two pouch-like glands behind the bladder that produce a fluid that provides sperm with an energy source that helps them move. The fluid from the seminal vesicles makes up most of the volume of ejaculatory fluid.

Sphincter—A round muscle that opens and closes to let fluid or other matter pass into or out of an organ, for example, sphincter muscles keep the bladder closed until it is time to urinate.

Testosterone—The male hormone responsible for sexual desire and for regulating a number of body functions.

Transrectal ultrasonography—A probe is inserted into the rectum to direct sound waves to produce an image of the prostate.

Transurethral resection of the prostate (TURP)—An instrument with a small loop of wire on the end is inserted in the end of the penis and threaded through the urethra. The wire is heated and cuts out obstructing tissue in the prostate. This procedure helps relieve symptoms of difficult urination or swollen prostate. It is not a treatment for prostate cancer.

Tumor—Abnormal growths or masses of tissue are called tumors. Many are benign (noncancerous) and some are malignant (cancerous).

Tumor stage—This medical labeling system indicates how far prostate cancer has spread.

Urethra—The tube that carries urine from the bladder to the outside of the body. It is also the channel that carries semen.

Urinary incontinence—The inability to control urination. It can be a side effect of prostate cancer treatment.

Ultrasound—Also known as a sonogram, this technique bounces painless sound waves off organs to create an image of their structure and abnormalities.

Urologist—A doctor who specializes in diseases of the male reproductive system and urinary tract.

Watchful Waiting—Also called active surveillance, it involves monitoring slow-growing prostate cancer through regular checkups rather than immediately treating it.

My Story

Many wise people (they may or may not have had prostate cancer) have suggested that laughter is the best medicine, and it may be the major behavior that separates us from other beasts (hyenas don't count). So I keep smiling, laughing, and acting beastly. Snickering, giggling, guffawing, and smirking may count, too.

Now what? Well, there may be other available trials and I'll certainly look. Would I fit into another trial? Will it be harder now that I have completed three?

Why can't I find some magic beans and fairy dust now that I really need them?

Every morning I wake up and smell the coffee and then I drink a bunch of it, too. One of these days someone will discover the hitherto unknown cancer-fighting benefits of strong coffee.

And furthermore. I intend to run another marathon or two, hike in the desert, run a few more trails, drive my jeep places it shouldn't go, and travel to distant and exotic ports. Of course, this depends as much on social security and the stock market as it does on my health.

I dutifully keep track of the inexorable increase in my PSA every month or two—sometimes it even goes down a bit. I know the tests and x-rays and scans won't cure me, but they drive my health insurance provider crazy and I get some satisfaction from that. Some seemingly innocuous test may tell my doctors that something needs tending—maybe my blood count is too low or there is a tumor on a bone, or just *maybe I've experienced a miraculous cure or improvement. Look for my picture on the cover of some obscure medical journal if that happens (I'll be the old gray guy with the big smile).*

Because I can't predict my immediate future very well (long term is a lot easier—nobody lives forever), I'm making sure that every day includes doing at least one thing that I really want to do— as long as I have permission from my wife and it's not illegal (and the illegal part may actually be optional). Decide what makes you happy and then do it.

You never know what might happen—in an ironic and unexpected twist, my oncologist and I have just published a book! Cancer Clinical Trials. *You might want to check it out!*

And check out what's happening in the prostate cancer world on my Prostate Cancer Blog at:

www.axman-axman.blogspot.com

May the force be with you (and me)!

THE BEGINNING (not the end)

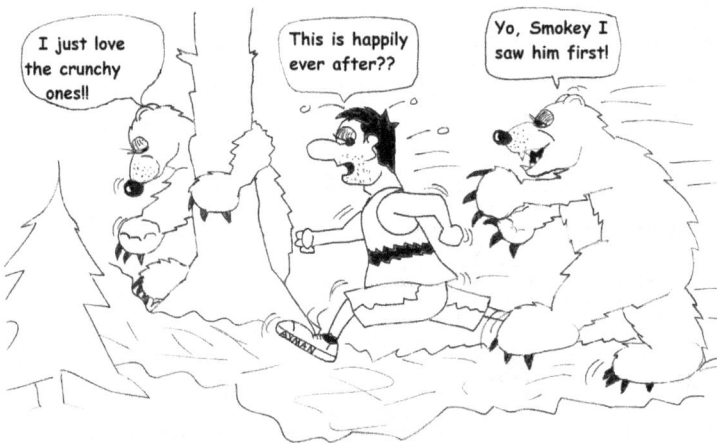

Index

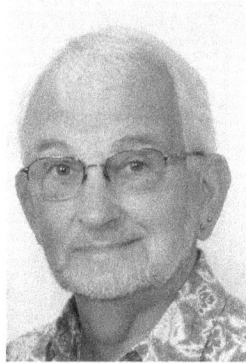

(More than you need to know) About the Author

Larry Axmaker is currently mostly retired after a 45-year career that included teaching, counseling, writing, and administration at all educational levels from elementary school through graduate school, private practice in Clinical Psychology, and more than a dozen years of writing, editing, and graphic art in health education and promotion. He is also solely to blame for all the cartoons in this book.

In addition, he has run more than 75 marathons and ultra-marathons, helped (a little) his wife, Carol, raise five children while living in various geographical locations, including Canada, Hawaii, Texas, and Oregon. He is currently trying (unsuccessfully) to keep up with his grandchildren.

He was diagnosed with prostate cancer in 2003 and has undergone both first line (surgery) and secondary (radiation) treatments originally designed to cure. Later on, he participated in clinical trials and took medications to slow the progression of his cancer. He is still slowing down, in more ways than one.

www.ingramcontent.com/pod-product-compliance
Lightning Source LLC
Chambersburg PA
CBHW060901280326
41934CB00007B/1135